DRUGS IN PRISON

Related titles:

Beta Copley and Barbara Forryan
Therapeutic Work with Children and Young People

Raymond Flannery
Preventing Youth Violence: A Guide for Parents, Teachers and Counsellors

Steve Gravett
Coping with Prison

Louise O'Connor, Denis O'Connor and Rachel Best
Drugs: Partnerships for Policy, Prevention and Education

J. Schulze and W. Wirth
Who Cares? Social Service Organizations and their Users

Drugs in Prison

A Practitioner's Guide to Penal Policy and Practice
in Her Majesty's Prison Service

STEVE GRAVETT

Continuum
London and New York

Continuum

The Tower Building
11 York Road
London
SE1 7NX

370 Lexington Avenue
New York
NY 10017–6503

First published 2000

British Library Cataloguing-in-Publication Data
A catalogue record for this book is available from the British Library.

ISBN 0-8264-5127-6 (hardback)
     0-8264-5129-2 (paperback)

Typeset by Paston PrePress Ltd, Beccles, Suffolk
Printed and bound in Great Britain by The Cromwell Press, Trowbridge, Wiltshire

Contents

	List of Charts and Tables	vi
	Foreword by Paddy Costall	vii
	Preface	ix
	Acknowledgements	xii
	How to Use this Book	xiii
	List of Abbreviations	xv
1	Dangerous Drugs	1
2	Prisons and Drug Misuse	22
3	Tackling Drugs in Prison	39
4	Drugs Prevention	51
5	Mandatory Drug Testing	63
6	Reducing Demand for Drugs	82
7	Drug Treatment Programmes	105
8	What Works?	127
9	Reviewing Performance	151
10	Planning for the Future	182
	Glossary	194
	Appendix I: Documents	196
	Appendix II: Addresses	199
	Index	203

List of Charts and Tables

Figure 1: The CARAT process flowchart   47
Figure 2: Notice to visitors document   54
Figure 3: Reducing the supply of drugs flowchart   57
Figure 4: Positive random test results chart   60
Figure 5: Prisoner's Consent to the Transfer of Information form   84
Figure 6: Flowchart of the CARAT process for a remand prisoner   87
Figure 7: Flowchart of the CARAT process for a sentenced prisoner   89
Figure 8: The compact on a voluntary testing unit   98
Figure 9: Flowchart of the treatment approach at HMP Downview   128
Figure 10: Flowchart of the treatment approach adopted at HMP Albany   129
Figure 11: Model of good practice: treatment strategy flowchart   137

Table 1: Punishment levels   78
Table 2: Reducing reconviction rates   149
Table 3: Overall rating assessment   183
Table 4: League tables   184
Table 5: Numerical overall rating assessment   184
Table 6: The scale of drug abuse   190

Foreword

When I was asked to write the Foreword for this book, I was pleased to accept for two reasons. First, I believe the subject is one of increasing importance and second, my involvement was another example of the increasingly close cooperation between staff from the Prison Service and those from external providers of services.

Since the publication of 'Drug Misuse in Prison' in 1995, the balance between the attempts to control the supply of drugs and the introduction of measures to increase access to treatment and reduce demand remains an issue to be resolved. Yet the willingness of those involved to engage in dialogue and work together towards common goals has been one positive outcome of the strategy to date.

The publication of the Government's ten-year strategy, 'Tackling Drugs to Build a Better Britain' (April 1998), was swiftly followed by the second Prison Service drug strategy, 'Tackling Drugs in Prison'. The strategy ensures that work with drug users in prisons is closely linked with interventions within the wider community. Interestingly, in that this is happening at a time when prisons generally are seeking to develop more solid links with the communities they serve, particularly with a view to strengthen the overall approach to tackling offending behaviour and reducing recidivism.

My own organization, Cranstoun Drug Services, has worked with drug users in prisons since 1982. One of our main tasks has been to assist prisoners to make and maintain links with external agencies, particularly in respect of post-release treatment and support. This approach has now been more widely adopted through the development of CARAT services throughout the Prison estate. (CARAT stands for Counselling, Assessment, Referral, Advice and Throughcare.) Latterly, Cranstoun has also become involved in the delivery of treatment programmes and staff training within a number of prisons, but brief interventions and a brokerage function on behalf of prisoners remain our core business.

The task of delivering drug services within prison presents additional challenges to similar provision outside. The recent massive development of prison-based services has exposed the lack of available, experienced practitioners to fill new posts. When staff are recruited, even those relatively experienced in service provision within the community, they require quality induction and support to enable them to adjust to work within the prison environment. A large part of this requires them acquiring knowledge of rules and systems, as well as developing an understanding of the culture of the prison(s) within which they work.

In this book, Steve Gravett covers, in a user-friendly way, most areas in which drug services would expect staff to be competent. I think the book also provides a way for prison staff to locate their work with drug users within their overall duties. His approach keeps jargon to a minimum and, where it is used, he provides explanations in plain English. The way the book is structured makes it accessible as a work of reference. The sections on drugs and their effects and on prison rules and adjudication processes are good examples of this.

Inevitably, any literature review for such a book must be selective, in view of the amount of works relating to prisons that have been produced. Steve has taken what I would describe as landmark publications, such as Woolf and Learmont, as well as using evidence from reports of HM Chief Inspector of Prisons, to chart progress in his chosen subject area. Some might take issue with his choice, but as a text for those new to the field, I think it describes adequately the framework within which developments have taken place. For those reading the book as an introduction to the work in prisons, the checklists at the end of each chapter provide a valuable aide-memoire to the learning process.

Another strength is the use of the case studies. I think an important aspect of these is that they demonstrate the ordinariness of most prisoners and highlight the common issues they present to workers from helping agencies. Many of the needs that emerge are related to relationships and situations outside the prison and thus point to the need for a more holistic approach. To use the language of community care, the provision of seamless services, provided within a multi-disciplinary framework.

Steve describes well the interventions now on offer within prisons for drug users. In particular, he describes the process by which prisoners can access the various interventions on offer. In this, examples of practice in various establishments are identified. If I were to have a criticism of this book, it would be that Steve fails to use examples of good practice that exist within HMP Camp Hill, where he is the Deputy Governor. Cranstoun staff have worked with prisoners in Camp Hill for many years and have generally met with a positive response from staff. My own involvement, principally with the prison management in the establishment and development of CARAT services, has been a rewarding experience. The support of senior management in any establishment is crucial to the sustainability of new services and I can say that this support is very real and effective within HMP Camp Hill.

Most of the book is devoted to description rather than opinion. Where opinions are expressed, I am sure they will not be universally accepted. This is a healthy position, provided those seeking to argue or criticize do so constructively, with the aim of taking issues forward. Also, some might say that the book fails to cover some aspects of the work, or that it doesn't cover them in sufficient depth. These may be legitimate criticisms, if Steve had claimed this to be a definitive text. I think any such criticisms should properly be met with an invitation to the critic to improve upon the contents herein and thus advance the creation of a more comprehensive catalogue of information for those working with drug users in prisons.

PADDY COSTALL
Director of Services
Cranstoun Drug Services

Preface

PROBATION SERVICE

STATEMENT OF PURPOSE

The Probation Service serves the courts and the public by:

- supervising offenders in the community;

- working with offenders, so that they lead law-abiding lives, in a way that minimises the risk to the public;

- safeguarding the welfare of children in family proceedings.

The Probation Service operates locally under probation committees or boards within a framework of national standards.

VISION

Aim

Effective execution of the sentences of the courts so as to reduce reoffending and protect the public.

Objectives

- Protect the public by holding those committed by the courts in a safe, decent and healthy environment.
- Reduce crime by providing constructive regimes which address offending behaviour, improve educational and work skills and promote law-abiding behaviour in custody and after release.

Principles

In understanding its work, the Prison Service will:

- Deal fairly, openly and humanely with prisoners and all others who come into contact with us.
- Encourage prisoners to address offending behaviour and respect others.
- Value and support each other's contribution.
- Promote equality of opportunity for all and combat discrimination wherever it occurs.
- Work constructively with criminal justice agencies and other organizations.
- Obtain best value from the resource available.

The Prison Service will also encourage prisoners to address offending behaviour and respect others. We will run our prisons in such a way that prisoners are motivated to use their time in custody positively.

We are committed to reducing re-offending through improved regimes for prisoners, by encouraging purposeful activity, through the improvement of educational and work skills, and through a wide range of offender treatment programmes.

A large number of prisoners use controlled drugs both inside and outside prison. We are determined to achieve a reduction in drug use amongst the prison population, through treatment programmes for drug users, as well as improving security.

The Prison Service VISION

Acknowledgements

My thanks to Martin Nary, the Director General of the Prison Service, who kindly gave me permission to write this book and reproduce several forms.

I am grateful for the cooperation of the Prison Service College Library at Newbold Revel, in particular Catherine Fell and Rebecca Mann. I appreciate the advice and guidance of Richard Rossington from the Drug Strategy Unit in Prison Service Headquarters.

Any views expressed in this book are solely those of the author and should not be interpreted as official Prison Service policy.

How to Use this Book

The Government's new drug strategy, 'Tackling Drugs to Build a Better Britain', and the Prison Service response, 'Tackling Drugs in Prison', herald a new era in drug penal policy. Major efforts are being made to resource this new policy on drug misuse. This strategy focuses on reducing the supply and demand for drugs in establishments, treatment programmes and seamless throughcare.

This comprehensive handbook covers mandatory drug testing, voluntary testing units, drug trafficking, active and passive drug dogs, treatment, counselling, health care and support services, together with the new CARAT service. An evaluation of how well the drugs policy is being implemented in establishments can be gauged from recent reports published by Her Majesty's Chief Inspector of Prisons. These are carefully analysed in the penultimate chapter. Case studies and checklists help bring the text alive and reinforce key learning points.

This user-friendly handbook complements my earlier book, *Coping With Prison* (1999), which is a comprehensive guide to penal policy and practice. *Drugs in Prison* concentrates on penal drugs policy and aims to be a comprehensive guide suitable for professional colleagues of all disciplines, students and prisoners alike. It contains valuable information for practitioners about drug misuse and focuses on current practice in a custodial setting. The pace of change in the penal field never ceases to amaze me. Inevitably some updating will be necessary as new legislation is introduced and policy is revised and amended in the light of experience.

The male gender has been used throughout for ease of expression and consistency. Unless mentioned specifically, policy and practice is identical in the case of female prisoners and female staff. A comprehensive index has been included to allow key words and sections of explanatory information to be found easily. The appendix of documents gives examples of forms referred to in the text, and the glossary explains more fully the meaning of important terminology.

This book is dedicated to the families of drug users, who suffer the terrible anguish of knowing that loved ones are ruining their lives, and know better than anyone how damaging drug taking can be to family life.

Finally, a special mention to anyone who has benefited from life saving drugs and, in particular, received chemotherapy. Only they really appreciate the miraculous difference the skilful use of modern drugs can make to the quality of life.

Any suggestions for improving this handbook will always be warmly welcomed by the author, who is now Deputy Governor of HMP Birmingham and can be contacted courtesy of the publisher.

STEVE GRAVETT

Autumn 2000

List of Abbreviations

6-MAN	6-monoacetylmorphine
ADD	Active Drug Detection
ADD	Attention Deficit Disorder
ADHD	Attention Deficit Hyperactivity Disorder
AIDS	Acquired Immune Deficiency Syndrome
BCG	Bacillus Calmete-Guérin
BoV	Board of Visitors
CARATs	Counselling, Assessment, Referral, Advice and Throughcare services
CCTV	closed circuit television
CNA	Certified Normal Accommodation
CPS	Crown Prosecution Service
CSR	Comprehensive Spending Review
DAAT	Drug and Alcohol Team
DAT	Drug Action Team
DCR	Discretionary Conditional Release
DRG	Drug Reference Group
DRU	Drug Rehabilitation Unit
E	ecstasy
EMIT	Enzyme Multiplied Immunoassay Technique
GNVQ	General National Vocational Qualification
GOAD	Good Order and Discipline
GCSE	General Certificate of Secondary Education
GS/MS	Gas Chromatography/Mass Spectrometry
H	heroin
HIV	Human Immunodeficiency Virus
HMCIP	Her Majesty's Chief Inspector of Prisons
HMSO	Her Majesty's Stationery Office
IEPS	Incentive and Earned Privilege System
KPI	Key Performance Indicator
LIDS	Local Inmate Data System
LSD	Lysergic acid diethylamide
MDMA	methylene-dioxy-mentyl-amphetamine
MDT	Mandatory Drug Testing

MRC	Medical Research Council
NAD	Nictinamide Adenine Dinucleotide
NHS	National Health Service
NVQ	National Vocational Qualification
OCA	Observation, Classification and Allocation
OSG	Officer Support Grade
PDD	passive dog detection
PEI	Physical Education Instructor
PIP	Primary Intervention Programme
ROTL	Release on Temporary Licence
RTU	Ready-To-Use
SAMHSA	Substance Abuse and Mental Health Services Administration
SARA	Substance Abuse Referral Unit
SIR	Security Information Report
SLA	Service Level Agreement
SMART	Specific, Measurable, Achievable, Realistic, Time-bounded
TB	Tuberculosis
THC	Tetrahydrocannabinol
UK	United Kingdom
VPU	Voluntary Prisoner Unit
VTU	Voluntary Testing Unit
XTC	ecstasy
YOI	Young Offenders Institution
YOTP	Young Offender Treatment Programme

CHAPTER 1

Dangerous Drugs

DEFINING DRUG MISUSE

Drug-taking is endemic in this country. The desire to take mood-altering stimulants appears to be irresistible. The everyday use of drugs has become part of our culture. Coffee, tea, cigarettes, wine, beer, whisky, sleeping pills and tranquillizers are drugs that can be taken legally. In prison, drug use is restricted to coffee, tea and cigarettes, and the temptation to acquire and misuse unlawful substances and drugs is considerable.

Effects on individuals

The effects of drugs on each individual vary enormously because there are so many unquantifiable factors to take into account. This means that over-generalizations as to 'cause and effect' can be misleading.

Consider the following factors:

- the amount taken;
- the previous history and tolerance of taking the substance;
- the expectations of the user;
- the physical surroundings;
- the reactions of other people present;
- the individual's body weight;
- whether a prisoner is pregnant;
- those with pre-existing psychotic tendencies.

Extreme results are possible with some individuals, and can be hazardous. For instance, someone taking cannabis, which is known to increase the heart rate slightly, could find the experience a painful one if he suffers from *angina pectoris*; and a psychotic person could be so badly affected by taking LSD or another powerful hallucinogen, that it tips him into the abyss of insanity.

Assessing risk

Taking any drug involves a certain degree of risk, despite exhaustive trials and prescribing by a qualified medical practitioner. Unfortunately, whether or not a drug is restricted legally is no guide as to its harmfulness.

The biggest danger facing drug users is that of overdosing. This can prove fatal, cause serious illness and increase the risk of accidents such as choking on vomit whilst unconscious. The risks associated with taking high doses of psychoactive drugs (those which affect the mind) over extended periods are that they distort perception, normal physical functioning and social relationships.

As the body develops more tolerance to a drug, the dosage increases and drug dependence is more likely to develop. This is accompanied by a wide range of symptoms which can last for several hours. Some of these symptoms are listed below:

- reduced desire for food;
- reduced libido;
- dulled reactions to pain;
- impaired walking ability;
- slower reactions;
- poor concentration.

Drugs and pregnancy

Doctors generally advise all pregnant women not to take any drugs, unless unavoidable. Taking illegal drugs during a pregnancy can damage the mother's health and directly affect the foetus. This risk is greatest in the first three months of pregnancy.

Despite the thalidomide tragedy, there has been a paucity of research into the effects of drugs on a foetus. However, heavy drug use by pregnant women is associated with:

- premature birth;
- low birth weight;
- stillbirth.

Babies born to drug-dependent mothers may become drug-dependent themselves and need medical assistance to avoid withdrawal problems.

Injecting risks

Injecting drugs is a high-risk activity. It is normally restricted to opiates, sedatives/ tranquillizers and stimulants like amphetamines/cocaine. An injected drug enters the bloodstream and is quickly carried to the brain resulting in an almost instantaneous effect. The rush associated with injecting drugs provides the user with a more intense experience than does taking them orally.

Injecting drugs under the skin or into the muscles provides a slower and less intense sensation than intravenous injection.

There are considerable risks attached to injecting drugs which include:

- overdosing;
- infections caused by sharing unsterilized needles;
- contracting Human Immunodeficiency Virus (HIV) and hepatitis B or C;
- gangrene and abscesses caused by missing the vein;
- health hazards resulting from injecting crushed tablets and substances not designed to be injected.

The adulteration risks

Mixing drugs and taking adulterated or impure substances amounts to taking a series of gambles.

Drugs sold or manufactured for the illicit market can vary considerably. Their strength is unknown and they may contain impurities which makes predicting the likely effects of such drugs difficult.

Mixing depressant drugs is extremely dangerous because the effect of each drug is cumulative, and a much lower dose of each drug can prove fatal. Benzodiazepines are potentially fatal if taken in sufficient quantities with alcohol.

Mixing drugs multiplies the chance of a harmful outcome. Cannabis is commonly mixed with other drugs either to boost or to suppress the effects of other drugs. Taken with alcohol, cannabis accentuates the depressant effect and loosens inhibitions. Ecstasy used with cannabis helps the individual relax and combats the tiredness and depression that usually follows when the effects of ecstasy wears off.

Drug misuse is a risky business. Apart from the high financial costs for the user of illegal drug-taking, the law takes a serious view of those who supply, possess and use drugs. Such misuse can lead to arrest, prosecution and, on conviction, the possibility of a custodial sentence.

DRUG LEGISLATION

The legal position regarding the availability of drugs in the UK is regulated by two sets of legislation.

The Medicines Act 1968 controls the manufacture and supply of all kinds of drugs. It classifies drugs into three categories:

- *Prescription only*
  Drugs that are prescribed by a doctor and obtained through a pharmacist working in a registered pharmacy.
- *Pharmacy medicines*
  Drugs sold without prescription but only through a pharmacist.

- *General sales list*
  Drugs that can be sold without a prescription by any shop, including a pharmacy.

The Misuse of Drugs Act 1971, which defines a controlled drug, is designed to prevent the non-medical use of certain drugs. This law clearly sets out several drug-related criminal offences that result in serious penalties on conviction:

- unlawful supply (including selling, sharing, exchanging and giving);
- intent to supply;
- trafficking offences (import and export);
- unlawful production;
- unlawful possession;
- allowing premises to be used to supply drugs.

This legislation divides controlled drugs into five schedules:

- schedule 1 drugs are the most restricted;
- schedule 2, 3 and 4 drugs can only be supplied for medical purposes on prescription;
- schedule 5 are drugs considered unlikely to be abused.

Schedule 5 drugs can be purchased from a pharmacist without a prescription, including some cough medicines, anti-diarrhoea products and mild painkillers.

Class A drugs

The potential penalties under the Misuse of Drugs Act 1971 are influenced by how harmful the drug is considered to be. Possession of a class A drug carries the most severe penalty, which can be up to seven years' imprisonment. Class A drugs include the following:

- the active ingredients in cannabis (schedule 1);
- hallucinogens (schedule 1);
- raw opium (schedule 1);
- cocoa leaf (schedule 1);
- opiates (heroin and morphine) (schedule 2);
- cocaine (schedule 2);
- phencyclidine (schedule 2);
- preparations which contain opium, morphine, cocaine and certain opioids (schedule 5);
- any class B drug used for injecting is treated as a class A drug.

Class B drugs

Possession of a class B drug carries a lower maximum penalty, but this can be up to five years' imprisonment. Class B drugs include:

- cannabis and cannabis resin/oil (schedule 1);
- strong stimulants such as amphetamines and methylphenidate (schedule 2);
- opiates such as codeine (schedule 2);
- methaqualone and mecloqualone (schedule 2);
- pentazocine (schedule 3);
- barbiturates except quinalbarbitone (schedule 3);
- mild opiates, opioids and non-injectable drugs which contain codeine (schedule 5).

Class C drugs

Class C drugs carry the lowest penalties, a maximum of two years' imprisonment for possession. Class C drugs include the following:

- dextropropoxyphene (schedule 2);
- weak stimulants such as diethypropion and phentermine (schedule 3);
- some sedatives and hypnotic drugs such as meprobamate (schedule 3);
- temazepam (schedule 3);
- rohypnol (schedule 3);
- benzodiazepine tranquillizers with the exception of temazepam (schedule 4);
- preparations which contain detropoxyphene designed to be taken orally (schedule 5).

The Drug Trafficking Act 1994

The Drug Trafficking Act 1994 makes it an offence to sell any article that enables someone to administer a controlled drug. It follows that cocaine kits are prohibited. The act also allows assets to be seized and income to be confiscated if it has come from the proceeds of drug-related crime.

UNDERSTANDING CONTROLLED DRUGS

This section examines the characteristics of a range of dangerous drugs that are commonly misused. It covers their legal status, recommended medical use, appearance, availability and effects, together with the risks associated with their use.

The eight groups of drugs selected are the same groups of drugs that are tested under mandatory drug testing (MDT) currently by the Medscreen Laboratory in London. Under MDT, a prisoner can be required to give a urine sample for testing, which is then sent away to Medscreen for analysis. A sample may be legally required providing the following criteria are met:

- on first reception into custody;
- on transfer from another establishment;
- as part of the risk assessment process;
- where it is suspected they have used a controlled drug;
- as part of the random testing programme.

Urine samples are subject to an initial screening test and, where necessary, a confirmation test is carried out to confirm the presence, or otherwise, of the following controlled drugs:

- cannabis;
- opiates;
- methadone;
- cocaine;
- amphetamines, including Ecstasy;
- benzodiazepines (tranquillizers);
- barbiturates;
- LSD (if requested by the sample taker).

CANNABIS

Name of drug
Cannabis sativa, which contains tetrahydrocannabinol (THC), herbal cannabis, cannabis resin and cannabis oil.

Drug group
Cannabis.

Slang names
Marijuana, draw, blow, weed, puff, shit, hash, hashish, ganja, grass, spiff, wacky backy, smoke, pot, oil, honey, skunk and northern lights.

Appearance
In its natural state, it is a dry, leafy substance and is called hemp. Most commonly, it is found as a solid, dark substance known as resin, or as a dark sticky greenish-brown oil.

Recommended medical use
A synthetic cannabinoid, THC is used for treating glaucoma. Also used to counteract the effects of nausea associated with cancer chemotherapy. The Medical Research Council (MRC) has commenced the first clinical trial to examine the health effects of

regularly using cannabis on patients suffering with multiple sclerosis. This three-year trial should determine to what extent cannabis offers effective relief to those suffering pain, muscle stiffness, sickness and tremors associated with the illness.

Legal status
Cannabis resin is a class B, schedule 1, controlled drug, but cannabis oil is a class A, schedule 1 drug.

How used
Cannabis is often rolled into a spiff or joint and taken with tobacco, or smoked in a special pipe. It can also be brewed in a drink or cooked and eaten. Whilst cooking cannabis makes the experience more intense, the effects are less predictable.

Duration of effects
The effect of smoking cannabis in small quantities is gradual and lasts for up to an hour. The effects can last for several hours when large doses are taken.

Availability
It is the most popular and widely available drug, particularly among young people in the 11–25 years age group. It is estimated that around five million people are using this drug in the UK.

Effects
- It acts as a mild sedative and reduces inhibitions.
- Users feel relaxed, drowsy and talkative.
- It slows reaction times and disturbs concentration.
- It can produce a craving for food known as 'having the munchies'.
- The user may have similar symptoms to someone who is under the influence of alcohol or sedatives, and may feel tired and apathetic, and lack energy and motivation.
- Users may experience an increased pulse rate, lower blood pressure, a dry mouth and bloodshot eyes.
- Heavy users may become anxious, confused, paranoid, experience panic attacks and, in extreme cases, have hallucinations.

Risks
- Smoking cannabis with tobacco may lead to the user becoming hooked on tobacco, which is perfectly legal.
- Smoking cannabis produces three times the tar content of tobacco.
- Long-term use can lead to respiratory problems, such as bronchitis, heart disease and an increase in the risks of lung cancer.
- A mentally ill user increases the risks of temporarily becoming mentally confused and suffering from delusions.
- Being 'stoned' increases the risks of having an accident if using machinery or driving a motor vehicle.

- Regular use during pregnancy can result in premature birth.
- Heavy use during pregnancy can result in a baby who suffers in the short term with tremors and distress, and is easily startled.
- The possibility of having a fatal overdose is virtually nil.

Cost

Herbal cannabis costs around £2–3 per gram and cannabis resin sells for about £3 per gram. Cannabis oil has a street value of approximately £15 per gram. It is a relatively inexpensive drug – for instance, as little as £1.50 worth of cannabis resin will make a couple of joints which can be shared with several others.

Treatment

Cannabis does not create any physical dependency in users and the withdrawal symptoms are fairly mild. It is frequently compared to tobacco, but tobacco, unlike cannabis, contains nicotine, a powerful, addictive and fast-acting drug. Tobacco also contributes to around 111,000 premature deaths and 2000 limb amputations in the UK each year, whereas there have been no reported deaths from a cannabis overdose.

OPIATES

Name of drug

Heroin, diacetylmorphine, diamorphine.

Drug group

Opiates are part of a group of drugs derived from the opium poppy. Opioids are the term used to describe synthetic drugs.

Slang names

Smack, junk, skag, horse, H, China white, brown, gear, jack.

Appearance

When pure, it is either a fluffy, white, fine powder or it occurs in small chunks. Street heroin, however, is often brownish-white.

Recommended medical use

Heroin is an effective painkilling drug that contains codeine and morphine. It is used to control severe pain in terminally ill patients.

Legal status

Heroin is a class A, schedule 2, drug. Doctors have to be licensed by the Home Office to prescribe heroin to registered addicts.

How used
Orally, sniffed, smoked and injected. 'Chasing the dragon' is when heroin powder is heated on tin foil and the fumes are smoked through a small tube.

Duration of effects
Between three and six hours, but this varies depending on the amount of drug taken and the extent of drug dependency.

Availability
Heroin is widely available illicitly. It can be purchased in a very dilute mixture as an over-the-counter medicine to treat coughs and diarrhoea.

Effects
- Small doses dilute the blood vessels giving a sensation of warmth and well-being.
- High doses make the user drowsy and relaxed.
- Excessive amounts which may lead to an overdose can result in coma and possible death.
- Heroin blocks any sensation of emotional and physical pain.
- When injecting, the user receives an intense sensation.
- The drug suppresses feelings of hunger, pain and worry.
- The initial reaction to taking heroin is nausea, dizziness and sickness.
- It depresses the nervous system and affects reflex functions such as coughing, breathing and heart rate.
- Heroin slows down bowel function, causing constipation.
- Sudden withdrawal causes severe discomfort for about five days, with influenza-like symptoms, muscular pain, aches, irritability, sweating and watery eyes.

Risks
- Heroin is an extremely addictive drug.
- Regular users develop a tolerance to the drug which means increasing amounts of heroin are necessary to maintain the same effect.
- Injecting carries with it the risk of infection from HIV/AIDS, septicaemia, hepatitis B and C, and abscesses; all these conditions are potentially life-threatening.
- Pregnant users need a maintenance dose of opiates until the baby is born, because withdrawal can kill the foetus.

Cost
Heroin which is 30–50 per cent pure costs between £50 and £80 per gram. It is often adulterated with glucose powder, chalk dust, flour or talcum powder, all of which have a similar appearance.

Treatment
'Cold turkey' is the expression used to describe the unpleasant side effects experienced by those undergoing withdrawal from heroin. Those not receiving medical super-vision take on a goose flesh appearance accompanied by shivering. After about six

hours, symptoms of anxiety and craving develop. These last about eight hours and are followed by perspiration, tears, a running nose and yawning. Within 24 hours, the pupils dilate, goose pimples appear, muscle tremors, hot and cold flushes, loss of appetite and painful muscles and bones develop. During the next stage, blood pressure, heart rate, temperature and breathing rate rise, and are accompanied by restlessness and insomnia. The final symptoms of withdrawal occur two days later and include vomiting (which exposes the user to suffocation by choking on their vomit) and diarrhoea (which causes severe dehydration).

Close medical supervision during the withdrawal phase is recommended. Methadone treatment can be prescribed as a substitute for heroin whilst the addict is gradually weaned off the drug. However, a common problem is that addiction to methadone replaces heroin addiction.

Another option is to give the registered heroin addict a reduced maintenance dosage of heroin.

Joining a therapeutic group or becoming a member of a therapeutic community can be valuable, whilst in serious cases admission to a psychiatric hospital for psychotherapy may be necessary.

METHADONE

Name of drug
Methadone.

Drug group
Synthetic opiates.

Slang names
Physeptone, amps (if injected), linctus (if taken orally).

Appearance
Available in tablet form, in a solution, syrup, powder or in capsules.

Recommended medical use
It is used as a heroin substitute and analgesic.

Legal status
It is a class A, schedule 2, controlled drug, available only on prescription.

How used
It takes about 30 minutes to achieve the maximum effect with a standard dose of 8–10 mg.

Duration of effects
Between four and six hours.

Availability
Not widely available on the illicit market; mainly used on prescription as a treatment for heroin addiction.

Effects
- It has a less euphoric effect on the individual, allowing him to function socially if receiving a regular dose.
- Blocks the sensation of pain and dulls any emotional reactions to it.

Risks
- Methadone is a highly addictive, synthetic drug.
- Those undergoing treatment often find they become addicted to methadone instead of heroin.
- The death rate and level of crime committed by methadone addicts is significantly lower than with heroin addicts.

Cost
Methadone costs around £1 for 10 ml or, if purchased in ampoules of 25 ml, approximately £25 each unit.

Treatment
Treatment works on the principle that methadone is the lesser of two evils, and is used as a substitute for heroin, which is very dangerous and highly addictive. Methadone treatment involves gradually reducing the dose to the point where it can be discontinued.

COCAINE

Name of drug
Cocaine, hydrochloride, cocaine freebase.

Drug group
Cocaine

Slang names
Coke, Charlie, snow, ice, freebase, base, rock, wash, stone and crack (which is a purer, smokeable form of cocaine).

Appearance
An odourless, white, crystalline powder. It is also available in chunks or rocks.

Recommended medical use
It can be used as a local anaesthetic but is normally used to relieve severe pain.

Legal status
Cocaine is a class A, schedule 2, controlled drug which is available only on prescription. Doctors have to be licensed by the Home Office to prescribe cocaine for addicts.

How used
Cocaine can be snorted or sniffed through a tube. Some users inject it and run the associated risks of contracting HIV/AIDS, whilst others mix it with heroin. 'Freebasing' is when cocaine is smoked after the cocaine base has been separated from the acid hydrochloride.

Duration of effects
Between 30 minutes and two hours.

Availability
Cocaine is manufactured in Peru, Bolivia and Columbia, and imported into this country in the form of cocaine hydrochloride. It is usually mixed with glucose powder before being sold on the illicit market. Before 1904, the drink Coca-Cola owed some of its popularity to small quantities of cocaine added to the ingredients. Some tonic wines supplied in the nineteenth century to popes and royalty also contained the added ingredient cocaine.

Effects
It is a powerful stimulant which gives an initial feeling of euphoria, making the user feel alert and confident. Once the effects wear off, the initial feeling of well-being is replaced by tiredness and depression. Other side effects include restlessness, nausea, insomnia, weight loss and paranoia.

Risks
- It can cause heart problems and chest pains.
- Digestive disorders.
- Loss of sexual desire and libido.
- Snorting cocaine can cause permanent damage to the inside of the nose.
- Psychological dependence can occur.
- Heavy use can cause convulsions.
- Frequent doses lead to users feeling restless, confused and paranoid.
- Users may take a further dose to delay the 'come-down effect' that is experienced once the drug wears off.
- Mixing cocaine with certain other drugs can have disturbing and unpredictable results. Mixing it with heroin, when it is known as 'speedball', can boost the effect, resulting in a heroin overdose. Such is the potency of this combination.
- Overdosing is risky and the symptoms are tremors, convulsions, hallucinations and agitation. Users have died from overdosing.

Cost
Cocaine is more expensive than other stimulants and is sold at around 20–50 per cent purity for between £50 to £100 per gram. Crack is available around 80–90 per cent purity for £25 for 150 mg. A weekend user is likely to average $\frac{1}{4}$ gram, whereas a regular user may consume 1–2 grams on a daily basis.

Treatment
Whilst heavy users of cocaine do not experience unpleasant withdrawal effects, as is the case with heroin users, the withdrawal symptoms include hunger, fatigue and depression. Although the side effects can be unpleasant, they do not pose serious health risks to users.

AMPHETAMINES

Name of drug
Amphetamine sulphate, dexamphetamine, laevo-amphetamine, methyphenidate, methylamphetamine.

Drug group
Amphetamines.

Slang names
Speed, whizz, uppers, dexedrine, dexies, benzedrine, bennies, ritalin, rit.

Appearance
A crystalline powder (known as ice), which can be obtained as pills, capsules or in injectable form.

Recommended medical use
Dexamphetamine and methylamphetamine are used to treat narcolepsy, a sleeping disorder that causes excessive drowsiness. They are also used to treat hyperkinesia, a condition which causes the patient to experience muscular spasms. Amphetamines can also be used as a slimming aid because they act as an appetite depressant.

Legal status
Amphetamines are a class B, schedule 2, controlled drug, which is available only on prescription.

How used
Amphetamines are usually smoked, sniffed, 'dabbed' on a finger or dissolved into a drink, then swallowed. Amphetamine sulphate is often injected to get an intense high called 'speed' or 'splash'. Freebasing is becoming more widespread, which is when the basic amphetamine is separated (and used for injecting) from the acidic (sulphate) part.

Duration of effects
Between two and four hours.

Availability
Amphetamines originate from Europe but are widely available because they are also manufactured in the UK. Apart from cannabis, amphetamines are the most widely used stimulant on the illicit market. In the 1960s, they were popular with the Mods who took purple hearts.

Effects
- Acts on the central nervous system as a stimulant, making the user feel more alert and energetic.
- Increases energy levels, confidence and the ability to concentrate.
- Reduces the need for food and sleep.
- Causes mood swings and agitation which sometimes result in violent behaviour.
- Using high doses on a regular basis can result in visual and auditory hallucinations or delusions.

Risks
- Amphetamines increase blood pressure, make pupils dilate and the mouth dry.
- Increases urination and causes diarrhoea.
- A temporary form of paranoid psychosis can result, from which it can take months to recover.
- Psychological dependence is possible as tolerance to the drug develops. Heavy users need to increase the dosage to maintain the mood-enhancing effects.
- In exceptional cases, heavy use can result in a stroke.
- A serious depressive state can accompany the withdrawal of amphetamines.
- Speed users sometimes indulge in binges which last for several days and are followed by a crash. This leaves them totally exhausted and in a state of psychosis.
- An 'up and down' drug-taking cycle is common amongst speed users who take amphetamines, then barbiturates, followed by amphetamines. This kind of dependence makes it impossible for them to hold down a normal job.

Cost
Amphetamines are ten times cheaper than cocaine products. The powder is often heavily adulterated, most commonly with chalk, caffeine or glucose powder, resulting in the purity being as low as 10 per cent. Amphetamine powder sells for around £10–15 a gram, amphetamine base for about £10–25 a gram, and 'ice' or 'crystal' for approximately £25 a gram.

Treatment
Unless users take excessive doses, toxicity is rare. Although the side effects associated with withdrawal can leave the user lethargic, hungry and very depressed, medical assistance is not normally required.

HALLUCINOGENIC AMPHETAMINES

Name of drug
Ecstasy, methylene-dioxy-methyl-amphetamine (MDMA).

Drug group
Hallucinogenic amphetamine.

Slang names
E, Doves, XTC, disco biscuits, echoes, hug drug, burgers, Adam, Love Doses, fantasy, Californian Sunrise, dolphins, mitsubishis, rolexes.

Appearance
Available in small or large clear capsules, round tablets, white, flat tablets with bevelled edges and occasionally as a powder. It comes in many different colours, but mainly white, pink or yellow.

Recommended medical use
Originally developed as an appetite suppressant.

Legal status
Ecstasy is a class A drug.

How used
Usually swallowed as tablets or capsules.

Duration of effects
Between three and six hours.

Availability
Originally associated with Acid-House music and parties in the 1980s, but now widely available.

Effects
- Users have boundless energy which enables them to dance for hours.
- Sound, colour and emotions are experienced more intensely.
- The user feels wide awake, less inhibited, relaxed, mellow and calm.
- It affects the body's temperature control so that users experience nausea, sweating, a dry mouth and an increased heart rate.
- Some people experience stiffness in the arms, legs and the jaw for short periods.

Risks
- Taking ecstasy and dancing for lengthy periods in a hot hall increases the likelihood of overheating, dehydration and heatstroke. This risk can be reduced by taking non-alcoholic drinks every hour and cooling down on a regular basis.

- It is linked to liver and kidney problems and eating disorders such as anorexia.
- Taking Viagra with ecstasy increases the possibility of heart problems.
- Ecstasy can cause damage to the brain leading to depression later in life.
- Affects the body's immune system causing respiratory failure and, in extreme cases, death. Around 60 deaths are attributable to ecstasy in the UK during the last decade.
- Apart from pregnant women, those most at risk are people with mental health problems, high blood pressure, asthma, glaucoma and epilepsy.

Cost
£8–10 per tablet.

Treatment
Ecstasy does not cause physical and psychological dependence. No major hallucinogenic side effects occur, although some users have frightening experiences. After using ecstasy, it is common to feel tired and depressed for several days.

BENZODIAZEPINES

Name of drug
Diazepam, chlorodiazepoxide, lorazepam, oxazepam, nitrazepam, flurazepam, temazepam.

Drug group
Benzodiazepines.

Brand names
Valium, Librium, Ativan, Serenid, Mogadon, Dalmane, Normison.

Appearance
They are available as tablets or capsules.

Recommended medical use
Benzodiazepines are used to control anxiety and help insomniacs. They can also be used to treat sports injuries by reducing muscle spasms.

Legal status
Benzodiazepines are a class C, schedule 4, controlled drug, available only on prescription.

How used
They are swallowed as pills and capsules, or injected.

Duration of effects
Between four and eight hours.

Availability
They are freely available and are the most frequently prescribed drugs in the UK.

Effects
- They reduce mental alertness and inhibit clear thinking.
- Benzodiazepines cause drowsiness and lethargy.
- They offer relief from tension and anxiety by enabling the individual to remain calm and relaxed.
- They exaggerate emotional responses which can lead to unusual and aggressive behaviour.
- Tolerance develops fairly quickly, making them ineffective as sleeping pills in as little as two weeks and inappropriate as a treatment for anxiety after four months.
- If taken with other drugs, particularly alcohol, the user loses inhibitions and can appear very drunk.

Risks
- They are relatively safe compared to barbiturates and a significant number have to be taken for a fatal overdose.
- They can disguise and exacerbate depression.
- Injecting temazepam is very risky because the gel in the capsule solidifies in the veins and can result in gangrene and subsequent amputation of limbs.
- Those on a high dose experience mild withdrawal symptoms for about two to three weeks. These are insomnia, anxiety, tremor, irritability, headaches, nausea, vomiting and hypersensitivity.
- Users taking very high doses can experience mental confusion, fits and life-threatening convulsions when in withdrawal.
- It causes psychological dependence and encourages excessive usage.
- Mixing benzodiazepines with barbiturates or alcohol is dangerous and can easily lead to respiratory failure, unconsciousness or death.

Cost
Individual diazepam tablets fetch between about 50p and £1 each and temazepam tablets cost 40p for each 10 mg tablet.

Treatment
Where treatment has continued for several years, normal therapeutic doses result in mild withdrawal symptoms.

BARBITURATES

Name of drug
Quinalbarbitone, amylobarbitone, phenobarbitone, butobarbitone.

Drug group
Barbiturates.

Slang names
Downers, Barbs.

Brand names
Seconal, Tuinal, Nembutal, Soneryl, Amytal.

Appearance
Barbiturates are available as tablets and capsules.

Recommended medical use
They are prescribed in severe cases of insomnia and used as a sedative. Phenobarbitone is used as an anticonvulsant to treat epilepsy.

Legal status
Barbiturates are a class B, schedule 2, controlled drug which is available only on prescription.

How used
They are usually supplied as pills, coloured capsules, suppositories, ampoules or a soluble solution. Drug users often inject barbiturates or take them with alcohol. They are used to control the negative side effects of other drugs, in particular amphetamines.

Duration of effects
From one hour up to sixteen hours.

Availability
They are not as readily available as benzodiazepines, which are safer and more easily obtained.

Effects
- They depress the central nervous system and have a similar effect to alcohol, making the individual feel relaxed, sociable and good-humoured.
- Injecting barbiturates gives an immediate feeling of well-being and drowsiness.
- They can cause an unpredictable or extreme emotional response.
- A moderate to large dose causes incoherence and clumsiness, increasing the risk of having an accident.

Risks
- It is very easy to overdose with barbiturates since the fatal dose is close to the normal dose and as few as ten tablets can kill.
- Injecting barbiturates runs the risk of gangrene, septicaemia and HIV/AIDS infections.
- Regular users increase the risk of contracting bronchitis and pneumonia.
- Frequent users build up tolerance over time and this can develop into a strong physical dependency.
- Barbiturates are very dangerous if mixed with any other drugs, particularly opiate-type drugs and other depressants.
- Mixing barbiturates with alcohol increases the risk of overdosing.
- Elderly persons and anyone suffering with heart problems, respiratory difficulties, glaucoma, epilepsy, hydrothrodism or jaundice should avoid barbiturates.
- Pregnant women who take barbiturates late in the pregnancy may give birth to a baby who experiences withdrawal symptoms.

Cost
Not applicable since there is little demand for these drugs currently.

Treatment
The effects of withdrawal usually last about a week. A user who has been taking very high doses can develop complications and develop bronchitis, pneumonia and hypothermia, and can accidentally overdose when in a confused state.

LSD

Name of drug
Lysergic acid diethylamide, LSD.

Drug group
It is a synthetic hallucinogenic drug originating from a fungus called ergot which grows on rye.

Slang names
Acid, trips, tabs, blotters, dots, micro-dabs.

Appearance
A synthetic white powder which is made into tablets or capsules, absorbed on paper squares, card, gelatine sheets and sugar cubes. Most LSD comes on small pieces of card or paper with colourful designs on the front.

Recommended medical use
A hallucinogenic drug that was originally used during psychotherapy. Since 1973, it can only be used under licence by the Home Office for research purposes.

Legal status
It is a class A, schedule 1, controlled drug.

How used
LSD is usually impregnated into squares of blotting paper known as tabs which are dissolved in the mouth. It only takes a tiny amount of this psychedelic drug to have a major effect – for instance, enough LSD for a trip would be 75 micrograms.

Duration of effects
LSD usually takes effect half an hour after taking the drug, reaching maximum effect after two to six hours. It fades away after twelve hours.

Availability
It is widely available at raves and discos and is becoming nearly as popular as amphetamine sulphate. LSD is the second most popular drug after cannabis.

Effects
- LSD is a powerful hallucinogenic drug which has a major effect on the mind, stimulating the imagination and making the user feel intoxicated.
- A trip has several phases to it and can last from eight to twelve hours.
- The effects of a trip are influenced by the user's state of mind, the company and the location.
- Users lose all sense of time, and shapes take on distorted appearances.
- Colours take on very intense kaleidoscopic qualities and sounds become distorted.
- Every trip is a different experience and the effects are unpredictable.
- Users experience dilated pupils, increases in heart rate, blood pressure, body temperature, as well as headaches and vomiting.
- Emotional reactions include increased self awareness, feelings of ecstasy, mood changes and abnormal perceptions.
- A tolerance to LSD builds up very quickly, which makes further doses ineffective after three to four days' use.
- Physical dependence does not occur with LSD.

Risks
- Once the experience known as a trip starts, there is no way of stopping it.
- Bad trips usually happen when the user is feeling nervous, uncomfortable or anxious.
- A bad trip can make the user feel very frightened, paranoid and out of control.
- High doses of around 250 micrograms can cause psychosis, temporary insanity and acute psychiatric breakdown.
- Users experience flashbacks, which is where part of the original trip is briefly relived, sometimes weeks or months later.
- LSD can exacerbate existing conditions such as depression, anxiety and schizo-phrenia.

- Accidents can happen whilst hallucinating, and tasks requiring concentration, such as driving a motor vehicle, are very dangerous.

Cost
LSD tablets are cheap and cost between £3 and £5 each.

Treatment
There are no known dangers associated with long-term use and few users become psychologically dependent. Tolerance to LSD builds up within a few days, but abstinence does not cause withdrawal problems.

CHECKLIST

- What is drug misuse?
- Why does taking the same drug affect people differently?
- Are the risks associated with using class A drugs greater than other drugs?
- What is the biggest danger facing someone who is drug-dependent?
- How do drugs affect pregnant women?
- Identify the health risks associated with injecting drugs.
- How does mixing drugs increase the risks facing drug users?
- Why are illicit drugs adulterated with other substances?
- What is the definition of a controlled drug under the Misuse of Drugs Act 1971?
- Why are drugs classified as class A, class B and class C?
- For which drugs does the laboratory test when a sample of urine is taken under mandatory drugs testing?
- Under what circumstances can a prisoner be required to provide a urine sample for drug testing?
- How is cannabis resin most commonly taken?
- What does 'chasing the dragon' mean?
- Who can benefit from methadone treatment?
- What does 'cold turkey' mean?
- Which soft drink originally included a controlled drug in the ingredients?
- What is 'freebasing'?
- How are amphetamines used to treat patients?
- What is the most frequently prescribed drug group in the UK?
- Why is it easier to overdose on barbiturates than on any other drug?
- Which class A hallucinogenic drug was originally used during psychotherapy?
- What is a 'bad trip'?

CHAPTER 2

Prisons and Drug Misuse

THE NATIONAL STRATEGY

In October 1994, the Government published a consultation document in the form of a Green Paper entitled 'Tackling Drugs Together' (HMSO). This was the product of the Government reviewing its strategy for tackling drug misuse in the UK.

In April 1998, the Government published a White Paper entitled 'Tackling Drugs to Build a Better Britain', which is their ten-year strategy to tackle drugs. It has four main aims, which are as follows:

1. *To help young people resist drug misuse in order to achieve their full potential in society.*
2. *To protect our communities from drug-related anti-social and criminal behaviour.*
3. *To enable people with drug problems to overcome them and live healthy and crime-free lives.*
4. *To stifle the availability of illegal drugs on our streets.*

The strategy document puts the causes of drug misuse in context and links problematic drug misuse with social problems such as unemployment, homelessness and social exclusion. Family and peer group pressures are major influences on individuals, although in the final analysis it is the individual who decides whether to take drugs or resist the pressure. Some youngsters are more likely to experiment and become drug-dependent; those most at risk are truants, young offenders, children in care and homeless young people.

The availability of drugs is increasing as worldwide production of drugs, such as cannabis, heroin and cocaine, is expanding, and trafficking routes becoming more ingenious and sophisticated. Although the amount of drugs being confiscated is rising, and the number of convictions in the courts increasing, prices on the streets remain constant. There is some evidence that the supply of drugs is outweighing demand, that purity levels are increasing, and that some drugs are being stock-piled.

Drug use is widespread amongst the working population, with estimates that one in ten adults (aged between 16 and 59) are drug users. The situation amongst school children is even more alarming and is getting worse. Children are experimenting with drugs at a younger age then ever before, as the following shows:

- *one in twelve* 12 year olds have tried drugs at least once;
- *one in three* 14 year olds have tried drugs at least once;
- *two in five* 16 year olds have tried drugs at least once;
- *one in five* 16 year olds have used drugs in the past month.

The health risks associated with drug misuse are significant and are exacerbated whenever a cocktail of illegal substances is taken. The consequences include an increased risk of lung diseases, liver damage, psychiatric conditions, schizophrenia, seizures, shock, coma and death. The number of drugs-related deaths continues to rise, with 1805 attributable deaths reported in 1995.

The strong link between drugs and crime is borne out by research. Half of those arrested reported illegal incomes which were 200–300 per cent higher than those arrested for reasons that were not drug-related. The Government estimates the social and economic costs of drug-related crime to be in the region of £3–4 billion a year. In addition, an estimated £1.4 billion is spent on drug-related public services each year (1997–8 figures), with 62 per cent of that figure spent on enforcement: the police; the Probation Service; the courts and the Prison Service.

This new strategy is comprehensive and examines significant research which provides useful evidence for tackling the drug problem. It places a strong emphasis on evidence-based research and on evaluating these findings to discover what works. The findings are encouraging and support the belief that much can be done to address the drug problem and help individuals, particularly young people, to resist the pressure and temptation to misuse drugs.

The first aim
To help young people resist drug misuse and so achieve their full potential in society, the national strategy focuses on drug education and prevention within and without schools, and drugs publicity and information campaigns.

The second aim
To protect communities from drug-related anti-social and criminal behaviour, the strategy examines linking the criminal justice system and treatment interventions; police action against drug-related crime and drug dealers; community involvement; drugs and the environment; drugs in clubs and pubs; drugs in the workplace and drugs and driving.

The third aim
To enable young people with drug problems to overcome them and live healthy and crime-free lives, the strategy explores the following:

- making contact with problem drug misusers;
- treatment for young drug misusers;
- outreach services;
- crisis intervention;
- prisons;

- the aims of treatment;
- harm reduction;
- detoxification and substitute prescribing;
- rehabilitation;
- meeting the needs of specific groups;
- race and drug misuse;
- mental health and drug misuse;
- pregnancy and drug misuse;
- women and drug misuse.

The fourth aim
To stifle the availability of illegal drugs on our streets, the national strategy examines intelligence-led and partnership approaches, including diplomatic and liaison activity in source and transit countries; the supply of drugs to and into the UK; supply and distribution networks within the UK; suppliers and dealers at local and street level; and the supply of drugs in prisons.

The strategic role of the Prison Service

Many drug misusers will continue to enter the prison system despite the existence of pre-custody, community-based opportunities. The penal system can achieve positive change with inmates who have been involved in drug-related offending providing it makes available advice, guidance, support and a range of different rehabilitative programmes.

Although treatment programmes in prison are a relatively new development, research shows that well managed programmes can have a major impact on reducing drug use in custody and on release. The key to successful programmes is using professionally qualified staff who have clear objectives and sound methodologies. The programmes need to be fully integrated into the prison regime with proper through-care plans devised to ensure that consistent and ongoing care in the community takes place following release.

A challenging target for the Prison Service is to reduce the amount of drugs visitors bring into establishments. Prisoners put considerable pressure on their visitors to bring in illegal substances, partly because they are being bullied, are afraid of reprisals from the wing-based drug dealers, or are plain greedy. During 1997, the police arrested 1183 visitors for drug-related offences. In 1998 it was 1114 and in 1999 had reduced to 828. In the first quarter of 2000, the number arrested had fallen to 112.

The following measures have proved to be effective in reducing the level of drugs entering prisons:

- the use of CCTV in visiting areas and in Visitor Centres;
- the use of passive drug dogs outside visit rooms;
- improved searching techniques for prisoners and their visitors;
- the use of closed visits for prisoners known to be drug users (closed visits take place in a cubicle where no physical contact is possible);

- displaying posters advising how many visitors have been convicted of smuggling drugs into the establishment;
- good liaison and sharing of intelligence between prisons and the police about prisoners and their visitors;
- confidential telephone hot lines to enable prisoners and visitors to provide information to establishment security departments;
- staff training for those helping in Visitor Centres to advise visitors under pressure against attempting to smuggle in drugs;
- amnesty bins for visitors to get rid of drugs rather than risk taking them into the establishment.

MONITORING PROGRESS

The first annual report by the UK Anti-Drugs Coordinator on the White Paper 'Tackling Drugs to Build a Better Britain', published 1999, highlights significant links between drug use and crime. It identifies that there is growing evidence that drug treatment works, but reveals that the availability of effective treatment services is failing to meet demand.

The report states that more money is being made available through the criminal justice system but there is concern that this money is spent on treatment facilities for the community as a whole, and that the Probation and Prison Services do not become protective of the money allocated to them, particularly in the historical context of a paucity of funding.

The author of the report believes that there is a public misconception that the Prison Service does not care and is ambivalent about the use of drugs in prison. He is finding that establishments are committed to the new prison strategy and can produce evidence that there is a significant reduction in the number of inmates testing positive for drugs. In addition, he draws attention to an increasing number of visitors being punished for possession of drugs and attempting to smuggle drugs into penal establishments.

Commenting on the newly published Prison Service drug strategy, he highlights its commitment to setting up a drug treatment service framework called CARATs – Counselling, Assessment, Referral, Advice and Throughcare Service – together with the development of more rehabilitation programmes. These have risen from 18 which existed before the strategy to a total of 48 programmes currently.

The Home Secretary's announcement in January 1999 to clamp down on visitors and prisoners involved in smuggling drugs into penal establishments is welcomed. This was accompanied by new powers to ban visitors who are caught or suspected of smuggling drugs.

Performance targets for 2005 and 2008

There are several national targets in the Anti-Drugs Coordinator's report that impact on the Prison Service. The overall aim is to create a healthy and confident society, increasingly free from the harm caused by the misuse of drugs. This is to be achieved by:

1. increasing the participation of problem drug users, including prisoners, in drug treatment programmes which have a positive impact on health and crime – by 100 per cent by 2008 and by 66 per cent by 2005;
2. putting in place more high quality treatment programmes and establishing CARATs as the basic treatment framework for prisoners by April 2000 (achieved);
3. ensuring that the CARAT service caseload reaches 20,000 by 2002;
4. providing 30 additional prison-based rehabilitation programmes by 2002;
5. enabling 5000 prisoners a year to complete treatment programmes by 2002;
6. improving security procedures in prisons to detect drug smuggling by April 2000. These measures include the following:
    (a) more drug detection dogs trained and deployed (achieved);
    (b) more CCTV in prison visits areas (achieved);
    (c) obtaining better intelligence concerning supply routes and the availability of drugs to prisoners;
    (d) measures to discourage families from smuggling drugs into establishments.

THE ROLE OF DRUG ACTION TEAMS (DATs)

The Government's Green Paper 'Tackling Drugs Together' (October 1994) established a number of principles for the effective coordination and delivery of the national strategy. These recommendations are based on the principles contained in the report 'Across the Divide' (produced by Roger Howard Associates in 1993 for the Department of Health) and stress the importance of multi-agency working; clear lines of accountability by one local agency to central Government; not tinkering with what works well already; a comprehensive geographical coverage based on identifiable local communities and involving very senior personnel from each organization.

Drug Action Teams

The crucial role of Drug Action Teams (known as Drug and Alcohol Action Teams – DAATs – in Wales) is to plan and deliver locally the strategy incorporated into the White Paper 'Tackling Drugs to Build a Better Britain'. The overall responsibility for coordinating this strategy lies with the Minister for the Cabinet Office.

The Government set up Drug Action Teams (DATs) in each district health authority area, with representation from the National Health Service (NHS), the local authority, education, police, probation and the Prison Service. The teams work at grass roots level with local communities and encourage a systematic approach to local planning. They use a standard template to assess and evaluate what is being done to combat drugs.

The remit of each Drug Action Team is:

- to tackle the drug problem in its district;
- to ensure the policies and practice of local agencies are in line with each other;
- to progress the Government's drug strategy by developing a local action plan.

Delivering the strategy locally

All local agencies are encouraged to work together to plan an effective programme of activity against drugs which supports the national strategy and its four main aims (refer back to p. 22 for these in full).

Under the first objective, *Young People*, DATs assess what action is being taken to increase the availability of information to vulnerable groups and services in the community. This includes young offenders and the children of drug-misusing parents.

Under the second objective, *Communities*, DATs form partnerships with Youth Offending Teams to address drug-related crime. The aim is to identify the number of drug-using offenders being referred for treatment.

Under the third objective, *Treatment*, DATs aim to improve the effectiveness and availability of local treatment services. Current provision is inconsistent and insufficient, with groups like women, ethnic minorities and young people under-represented, despite the availability of good quality information and advice services in the community.

Under the fourth objective, *Availability*, DATs are trying to put in place better systems for the accurate gathering and processing of data. This will enable them to prioritize and coordinate multi-agency working effectively.

The Drug Action Team agenda

The agenda set by the Government means that local agencies need to work towards reducing the use by young people under the age of 25 of the most dangerous drugs, namely crack, cocaine and heroin. Feeding a drug habit has a major effect on crime. For instance, an income of £10–20,000 a year is needed to feed a heroin or crack habit, and this is earned illegally, mostly through burglary and theft.

National targets for reducing the use of class A drugs by young people are a 25 per cent reduction within five years, and a 50 per cent reduction within ten years. By 2002, all DATs should have comprehensive and effective programmes using a life-skills approach, operating in all schools, the youth service, further education colleges and the community.

Health authorities are expected to:

- ensure a greater uptake of hepatitis B vaccination;
- assess the treatment needs of young drug misusers, in conjunction with the Youth Offender Teams, and address their identified needs;
- produce an action plan which meets local demand for detoxification and therapeutic programmes;

- arrange appropriate training for GPs and primary care teams;
- establish a maximum waiting time for those referred for drug treatment services.

DATs have a crucial role to play in the delivery of effective programmes to combat drugs in both the community and penal establishments. The Prison Service policy, 'Tackling Drugs in Prison', recognizes the importance of working closely with DATs and of ensuring that an effective partnership is established with other statutory and voluntary agencies in order to deliver the Government's national strategy. Each Prison Service Area Manager has appointed Area Drug Strategy Coordinators, who liaise regularly with all the Drug Action Teams in the area, and every prison is represented on the local Drug Action Team.

Drug Reference Groups (DRGs)

The publication 'Tackling Drugs Together' makes it a requirement to set up Drug Reference Groups (DRGs) to support Drug Action Teams in implementing the strategy. The main role of DRGs is to take forward the action agreed by the DAT, offer advice, and disseminate information about good practice and new initiatives.

DRGs are encouraged to widen their membership and representation so that all drug agencies active in the substance misuse field are included. They tend to have a wide-ranging membership which includes senior managers from the private and voluntary sectors, service user representatives, schools, colleges and general practice. The membership of a typical DRG may include:

- the purchasing manager from the *Social Services Department*;
- the director of a *Voluntary Drug Organization*;
- the chief environmental health officer from the *Environmental Health Department*;
- representatives from *service users and self-help groups*;
- school governors, head teachers and principals from colleges of further education, representing *education management*;
- general managers and marketing directors from the *business sector*;
- a policy officer from the *Government Training Council*;
- representatives from *housing organizations*;
- *general practitioners*;
- *pharmacists*;
- a manager from *HM Customs and Excise*;
- the manager of the *Youth Service*;
- a representative from the *Community Health Council*;
- a consultant from *specialist drug treatment*;
- the manager of *health promotion*;
- a coordinator from *health education*;
- the team leader of the *Drugs Prevention Initiative Team*.

DRGs have a role to play in supporting Drug Action Teams establish and develop close links with other DATs, Home Office Drugs Prevention Teams and other Government departments.

DAT action plans

'Tackling Drugs Together: A Practical Digest for Drug Action Teams' highlights examples of good practice. It examines closely the action plans compiled by the 105 DATs throughout the country, and stresses the need for DATs and DRGs to work closely together to ensure all available resources are used effectively to tackle drug problems. The publication emphasizes the need to be realistic about what can be achieved.

Many DAT action plans feature measures the Prison Service is taking to reduce the supply and use of drugs in prisons:

1. *Action to stop drugs entering prisons*
   - close cooperation and sharing of intelligence between the police and prison authorities;
   - increased perimeter security;
   - increased security on prison visits including the use of CCTV;
   - the searching of all visitors;
   - confidential drug telephone lines for prisoners and their families.
2. *Action to combat drug use in prisons*
   - the use of random searches in conjunction with mandatory drug testing;
   - conducting health-need assessment surveys;
   - providing drug awareness training for prison staff, aimed at persuading prisoners and their families not to smuggle drugs;
   - specialist counselling and support for prisoners with drug problems;
   - the inclusion of drug education in existing pre-release courses.
3. *Action to help prisoners on discharge*
   - making contact with the prisoner's home areas before release;
   - providing practical help after release, including finding suitable accommodation;
   - assisting prisoners to continue receiving support in community-based schemes;
   - making sure the demand for programmes can be met.

THE CHIEF INSPECTOR OF PRISONS' ASSESSMENT

The Annual Report of Her Majesty's Chief Inspector of Prisons (HMCIP) for 1998 applauds the new drug strategy for prisons 'Tackling Drugs in Prison', together with the national strategy, 'Tackling Drugs to Build a Better Britain'. The report particularly welcomes the additional funding, £76 million, that has been allocated under the Comprehensive Spending Review (CSR) over the next three years to tackle the problem.

The author of the report, Sir David Ramsbotham (HMCIP), acknowledges the difficulties inherent in evaluating these strategies in prisons and has co-opted several specialist drug inspectors to assist in the evaluation process. He highlights the approach adopted by the Area Manager in Kent as an example of good practice. Each establishment in Kent has been given a part to play in the area strategy and they all work together in a coordinated way. At HMP Elmley, a large local prison, each new reception is given a drug test and then either offered a place on a voluntary testing unit (VTU) or targeted for treatment, depending on the scale of his drug misuse. HMP Elmley liaises closely with the Kent Drug Action Team, Kent Police and a number of outside agencies, to ensure that throughcare is seamless when the inmate leaves prison. A separate programme targets dealers, making sure that they do not have contact with those dependent on drugs within the establishment.

The Inspector's concerns in his Annual Report centre around the lack of clear direction from Headquarters as to how each establishment should implement the strategies. He is particularly concerned about establishments catering for the needs of women and young offenders. This lack of a strategic approach can be seen in the way treatment programmes are delivered, but is also evident in the emphasis placed on preventing drugs getting into establishments. The way passive drug dogs are deployed illustrates this point – they have proved to be particularly effective in discouraging drugs from entering establishments, and governors are now strongly encouraged to seek CSR funding to pay for them.

The Chief Inspector notes that the Drug Strategy Unit in Headquarters has funded detoxification units in each local prison, but feels the detoxification programmes themselves are uncoordinated. At that time, he felt there was a lack of therapeutic drug treatment programmes to respond to identified need, and those available were offering entirely different programmes. He cites as examples the drug treatment wing at HMP Channings Wood, run by ADDACTION, and the unit at HMP Lindholme. This has now improved from three therapeutic drug treatment programmes to eight, including two for women.

He is emphatic that 'no subject attracts greater media attention in prisons than drugs, particularly questions about how and why they can be got into such closed environments'.

DEATHS IN CUSTODY

Her Majesty's Chief Inspector of Prisons published a thematic review in 1999 called 'Suicide is Everyone's Concern'. This establishes a link between a previous history of substance abuse and self-inflicted deaths by prisoners in custody. It concludes: 'about three quarters of people who take their own lives in prison have a history of substance misuse'.

This statement should be contrasted with comparable figures for those in the community where only 1 per cent of self-inflicted deaths in the community have a drug-dependency history. Despite this, the Inspector concludes that the level of self-inflicted deaths in custody from those prisoners with a drug-related offence is lower than he expected.

In 1998, eight prisoners charged with a drug offence committed suicide in custody, compared with seven prisoners in 1997, and eight prisoners during 1996.

Single/multiple drug users

During 1997, a total of 68 self-inflicted deaths occurred. Sixty-nine per cent of those prisoners who committed suicide had a history of single or multiple drug misusing: 28 per cent were single drug misusers; 41 per cent were multiple drug misusers.

In 1996, 64 prisoners committed suicide in prison. Seventy-seven per cent of those suicides were by prisoners who had a history of misusing drugs: 38 per cent were single drug misusers; 39 per cent were multiple drug misusers.

The drug misuser profile

An examination of the available data suggests that a profile of those drug users most likely to commit suicide in custody is beginning to emerge:

- white, male, adult prisoners;
- users with a history of taking opiates and/or cannabis;
- prisoners held in a local prison on remand;
- those with previous custodial experience.

Death occurs during the first month of being in custody, and the highest period of risk is the first week, with 10 per cent of all suicides occurring within the first 24 hours of custody.

Much of the data analysed is inconclusive with no particular pattern evident. However, the cause of death is sadly more predictable. It is death by hanging from a single-cell window, using bedding or clothing as a ligature.

EVIDENCE FROM PRISONERS

The inquiries into the escapes of Category A prisoners in 1995 were published in a paper known as the Learmont Report. This reported renewed security arrangements and included much evidence from prisoners. Several inmates told the Learmont inquiry team that drugs are the root cause of many problems in prison. Their availability causes concern to many inmates because the level of intimidation, bullying and assaults often has a direct link with drug abuse. Drug users put pressure on their visitors and those temporarily released on licence to smuggle in drugs to keep their habit going. Often, users build up debts with their suppliers. When this occurs, repaying these favours in order to pay off their debts may mean getting involved in carrying out assaults on other prisoners or applying pressure on their families.

In addition, some inmates had told the inquiry team they had seen over 40 people sharing the same needle.

The Learmont Report highlighted how phonecards are regularly used as currency for purchasing drugs, for gambling, for trading or for paying off debts.

The Report of an Inquiry by Her Majesty's Chief Inspector of Prisons into the Disturbance at HMP Wymott on 6th September 1993 found evidence of bullying, intimidation, regular assaults, widespread vandalism, a gangland culture and drug problems. Drug-taking was undermining the regime and threatening the safety of other inmates.

Following the HMCIP report on HMP Lincoln in 1997, there were lurid press reports of a reign of terror at a high-security jail which had reduced one wing to a 'no-go area'. It was claimed that prison officers were afraid to patrol and that bullies, thugs and drug dealers were able to roam freely. Usage was reported to be widespread, and a former inmate interviewed on BBC radio claimed the place was awash with drugs – providing you had the money, any drug was obtainable.

The same year, a prisoner at HMP Long Lartin, serving twenty years for a drug offence, claimed in a newspaper article that wild drug parties had been a regular nightly occurrence. He told how prison officers turned a blind eye to the smoking of cannabis, how smuggling drugs was easy because visitors were only superficially searched and strip searches for prisoners were a rarity. He claimed that since mandatory drug testing and differential regimes had been introduced, the effect had been dramatic: prisoners were randomly required to give urine samples for testing, and refusal or evidence of drugs in their body led to additional days added to their sentence. Life inside had been made intolerable now that visitors were searched, the use of passive drug dogs had begun, CCTV surveillance was in visits rooms, closed visits were enforced for acting suspiciously or trying to smuggle drugs through visits, and one was placed on the basic regime for refusing to work.

The prisoners' perspective

The All Party Parliamentary Drug Misuse Group became increasingly alarmed about press reports that prisoners were switching from soft to hard drugs whilst inside, and stories of prisoners becoming hooked on drugs whilst in prison. They decided to review the position in 1998 and spoke to a small sample of ex-prisoners who told them the following:

1. There is a huge market for drugs in prisons.
2. The lack of constructive activity in many prisons, as a result of financial cutbacks, has led to more prisoners turning to drugs as something to do.
3. Medical help for drug-dependent users is very sparse, the system is unsympathetic, and some people receive no help at all.
4. Prisoners run into debt, and family and friends are intimidated into bringing drugs into prison.
5. There is a considerable amount of violence, intimidation and bullying directly associated with drugs.
6. Many prisoners are switching from cannabis to harder drugs to avoid being detected under random mandatory drug testing. (This has since been researched and is not borne out by mandatory drug testing figures.)

7. Drug testing rarely occurs at weekends which allows prisoners to use opiates with impunity on Friday nights. (This has now been addressed and weekend testing takes place.)
8. Voluntary testing units (known as drug-free wings) are being abused by some prisoners who engineer a move to such wings in order to use drugs in safety.

RESEARCH FINDINGS

The Home Office commissioned the Oxford Centre for Criminological Research to evaluate what impact mandatory drug testing (MDT) was having on drug misuse in establishments. Their comprehensive study was published in 1998. To reflect a range of custodial settings, sentence length, gender and ages, they selected five different establishments: a Category C trainer; a Young Offender's Institution; a local prison; a dispersal prison and a women's prison.

The aim was to assess prisoners' experiences of MDT, examine whether the level of their drug use had changed, and gauge if their pattern of drug taking had changed.

They found cannabis and heroin were the most widely used drugs in prison. Seventy-five per cent of the prisoners admitted smoking cannabis and 40 per cent admitted taking heroin or misusing prescribed drugs in prison. A disturbing finding was that 20 per cent of the prisoners in the sample claimed that their first experience of using heroin was in custody. Most prisoners admitted a willingness to experiment with drugs whilst in custody, although in many cases, particularly of those under the age of 21, regular drug-taking was part of their normal lifestyle in the community.

Prisoner views on MDT

Prisoners were asked to comment on the impact mandatory drug testing was having on their behaviour:

- 48 per cent reported no change in their pattern of drug use;
- 27 per cent claimed MDT prompted them to stop using drugs;
- 25 per cent have reduced or modified their usage of drugs.

The degree to which prisoners were influenced by mandatory drug testing was dependent on several factors:

(a) their assessment of the likelihood of being detected and punished;
(b) how motivated they were to change their lifestyle;
(c) their perception of whether drug testing is a fair policy.

Two thirds of prisoners believed drug testing is an attempt by the authorities to restrict the use of cannabis in penal establishments. Over 80 per cent of prisoners did not believe cannabis is harmful and thought its use should be condoned.

Risks and consequences

Prisoners believe the likelihood of being selected and detected on the MDT programme is slim. They understand the stated target for random testing is 10 per cent of the population each month, but are aware many establishments cannot meet that quota and calculate the risks accordingly. A significant proportion (33 per cent) believe it is easy to get around the test, possibly by adulterating the sample in some way.

Prisoners who are tested on reasonable suspicion or for the purpose of a risk assessment are more concerned about the likelihood of being detected. They are far more inclined than those undergoing random testing to change their behaviour and improve their chances of being considered favourably for temporary release, parole or a progressive transfer.

Overall, mandatory drug testing has increased the risks of detection associated with drug taking and this has resulted in a decrease in the recreational use of cannabis. Most prisoners disagree with drug testing for cannabis, feeling it should be restricted to class A drugs. They consider the Prison Service has the punishment and treatment issues out of balance, and think that MDT has not improved the prospects of those prisoners who need help receiving treatment.

CONCLUSIONS

1. Drug testing is an expensive initiative. The cost of 'added days' arising from punishments for testing positive is equivalent to 360 prisoner years per annum, making an annual cost of £7m.
2. Twenty per cent of prisoners claim not to use drugs in prison.
3. MDT has a deterrent effect on about 50 per cent of all prisoners who are drug users.
4. Twenty-five per cent of users claim to have stopped using drugs completely.
5. Fifteen per cent claim to have reduced their consumption of drugs in prison.
6. Six per cent claim to have altered their pattern of drug misuse and now take less cannabis whilst continuing to use heroin.
7. Four per cent claim to have tried heroin for the first time in custody and have switched from using cannabis.

THE POLITICAL DIMENSION

Ministers believe the Prison Service approach to tackling drugs has to complement and be entirely consistent with the national strategy detailed in the White Paper 'Tackling Drugs to Build a Better Britain'. The new Prison Service drug strategy, 'Tackling Drugs in Prison', builds on three existing objectives: to reduce supply; to treat addiction and to minimize health risks.

The lessons from research are that the balance between random testing and targeted testing needs to be adjusted and this has been acted upon. The approach needs to shift towards targeting prisoners whose behaviour attracts suspicion, conducting risk assessments and encouraging voluntary testing. This allows Governors to challenge more prisoners about their drug taking and give them an opportunity to address their drug habit. In the case of young offenders, who are heavily involved in taking cannabis, the priority is to prevent them sliding into hard drug use.

Zero tolerance

Politicians are adamant that there is no softening in their approach to tackling drugs in prisons. They advocate a policy of zero tolerance towards drug-taking. Drug testing is a key weapon that needs to be concentrated on persistent offenders and those keen to stop their dependence on drugs.

Ministers believe that dealers and users of hard drugs should be tackled firmly because their behaviour undermines good order and discipline (GOAD) within establishments, and their anti-social activity damages other prisoners' prospects. They want Governors to differentiate more sharply in the punishments they award between users and dealers, and between drugs that are more harmful than others. They point out that the law makes this distinction in the Misuse of Drugs Act 1971 and want the Prison Service to reflect this in the advice issued to Governors conducting adjudications on prisoners.

Breaking the habit

Ministers want more prisoners to have an opportunity to break their drug dependency or addiction habit. This means allowing more prisoners access to voluntary testing schemes so they can remain drug-free. Coupled with the introduction of more voluntary testing units (VTUs) is the further development of more effective treatment programmes. They appreciate that external community drug agencies have expertise and experience in this area that many prison staff do not possess. Other key actions ministers wished to see taken, and which have been implemented, are more provisions for drug education, particularly for young offenders; improvements to existing throughcare arrangements; and the introduction of a prison area coordinator in each area.

COMBATING DRUGS IN PRISON

In their report 'Prisons and Drug Misuse' (July 1998), the All Party Parliamentary Drug Misuse Group endorsed the recommendation of the Advisory Council on the Misuse of Drugs, which stated 'that measures to tackle supply, demand, and harm reduction should be built into the routine planning policies and practice of each prison'.

Reducing supply

The report recommended that the Prison Service introduce national guidelines for reducing the supply of drugs into prisons. Every prison should supplement its existing security procedures with the following:

- a sniffer dog;
- a visiting centre with makes drug smuggling very difficult but provides a relaxed environment for law-abiding visitors;
- up-to-date screening equipment capable of detecting drugs.

Reducing demand

The report endorses an approach, particularly for young offenders, which counters the notion that drug-taking is an attractive alternative to boredom and inactivity in prison. It advocates providing an attractive regime comprising education, training courses, work and work experience placements.

Other identifiable ways to reduce the demand for drugs in prison is to provide establishments with drug-testing facilities and the capability to process urine samples rapidly, and introduce voluntary testing units which offer prisoners the option of living in a drug-free environment.

Reducing harm

The Drugs Misuse Group suggests the Prison Service and the Department of Health both develop a national harm reduction programme. It makes the following specific recommendations:

- routine screening for HIV, hepatitis B and C;
- anonymous sampling of all prisoners to assess the scale of the problem;
- introduction of needle exchange schemes;
- availability of sterilizing tablets to all prisoners;
- a targeted drug-testing programme which includes weekend testing.

Improving treatment

The Drug Misuse Group recommends that establishments introduce effective screening processes to identify prisoners with potential drug problems on first reception. They recognize there is a serious shortfall in the number of effective drug treatment programmes available in prisons, but believe the specific needs of remand prisoners, those serving short sentences, women and young offenders should be addressed.

The report highlights the need for seamless throughcare for prisoners who have completed a drug treatment programme, and argues that it is counterproductive to discharge any prisoners without addressing their accommodation and employment needs.

Several training needs are identified and the following are advocated:

* more accredited drug training for prison staff;
* more training for judges and magistrates about drugs misuse;
* examples of good practice are disseminated in a systematic way throughout the Prison Service.

CASE STUDY

John: Adult offender

John has a history of polydrug use, including three years using opiates (heroin) and crack. His involvement with drugs commenced as a teenager with cannabis resin and he has been involved ever since. He has sought help from a community-based drug agency for his heroin dependency and has received group work and counselling in the past.

Twelve months ago the courts imposed a probation order with a condition that he attend a drug treatment programme. This resulted in a place being found for him in a residential rehabilitation programme which he completed successfully. John began to live a drug-free life in the community but relapsed and started to take drugs again, committing burglaries to support his habit. He was arrested and subsequently sentenced to two years' imprisonment.

His relationship with his common-law wife is in crisis. The eldest of their three children is in the care of the local authority and his wife is caring for their two other children, aged 3 years and 18 months, in a one-bedroom flat. Since John was sentenced, she has resumed regular contact by letter and telephone. She visits regularly and brings the two younger children with her once a month when she can get a lift from a friend.

CHECKLIST

- Identify the four aims contained in the national ten-year strategy, 'Tackling Drugs to Build a Better Britain'.
- What measures have proved to be effective in reducing the level of drugs entering prisons?
- The Prison Service drug strategy includes a drug treatment framework called CARATs. List the elements of the CARATs approach.
- What are the national targets set for the Prison Service to achieve by 2008?
- Describe the main role of a Drug Action Team.
- How does the work of a Drug Action Team support the stated aims contained in the national strategy?
- What is the main purpose of a Drug Reference Group?
- Where does the Chief Inspector of Prisons feel there is scope for improving the strategy 'Tackling Drugs in Prison'?
- Suggest a typical profile for a drug user in prison.
- Why is there a perception that some prisoners switch from using cannabis to hard drugs?
- What is mandatory drug testing?
- Why are some prisoners subject to drug testing as part of the risk assessment process?
- What are the three main aims of the Prison Service drug strategy 'Tackling Drugs in Prison'?
- How does a policy of zero tolerance towards drug-taking work in prison?
- What is the role of a voluntary testing unit?
- How can the supply of drugs entering prisons be reduced?
- Identify three effective measures that can reduce the demand for drugs in prisons.
- What does 'harm reduction' mean in relation to drug misuse?
- Explain the meaning of 'seamless throughcare'.

CHAPTER 3

Tackling Drugs in Prison

UNDERSTANDING THE PRISON SERVICE DRUG POLICY

In May 1998, the Prison Service launched a new drug strategy called 'Tackling Drugs in Prison', which complements the Government's national ten-year strategy 'Tackling Drugs to Build a Better Britain'. The former built on the framework document contained in 'Drug Misuse in Prison', published in April 1995.

This new strategy is constructed around the four aims contained in 'Tackling Drugs to Build a Better Britain' (detailed briefly in Chapter 2). They are as follows:

1. *To help young people resist drug misuse in order to achieve their full potential in society*
    (a) to control the supply and demand for drugs in custody;
    (b) to develop best practice in education about drug misuse, particularly for juveniles and young offenders, given that the peak age for drug misuse amongst prisoners is 23;
    (c) to provide the best in drug education in a supportive but disciplined environment for juveniles;
    (d) to develop constructive regimes for all inmates which provide an incentive to look ahead to a life without drugs;
    (e) to liaise closely with other agencies in the youth justice system and provide effective throughcare for juveniles and young offenders on release;
    (f) to examine the particular needs of female prisoners.
2. *To protect our communities from drug-related anti-social and criminal behaviour*
    (a) to target those who seek to profit from the misuse of drugs in prisons;
    (b) to develop a performance indicator which is based on action taken against suppliers and dealers;
    (c) to make anti-social drug-related activity a key criterion within establishment incentive and earned privilege schemes;
    (d) to encourage Governors to discriminate effectively within the disciplinary system between more and less harmful drug-related activity;
    (e) by conducting research to assess the effectiveness of prison-based intervention strategies, and their impact on reducing recidivism following release.

3. *To enable people with drug problems to overcome them and live healthy and crime-free lives*
   (a) to examine the adequacy and availability of resources for effective treatment interventions;
   (b) to appoint Area Drug Coordinators to conduct a needs analysis in each area and devise and cost strategies which give all inmates access to voluntary testing;
   (c) to improve the match between identified need and appropriate treatment provision;
   (d) to provide advice on setting up voluntary testing units together with a range of treatment opportunities suitable for offenders;
   (e) to reduce the number of random drug tests Governors are required to carry out in their establishments, and encourage a commensurate increase in the number of voluntary, repeat and targeted testing;
   (f) to ensure drug issues are effectively tackled in the sentence management and throughcare arrangement process;
   (g) to devise effective strategies to help short-term and remand prisoners, and increase the level of referrals to community-based agencies;
   (h) to work with the UK Anti-Drugs Coordinator and other agencies to develop agreed quality standards for effective practice, which covers assessment, interventions and relapse prevention;
   (i) to encourage close liaison between HIV and AIDS teams and those responsible for taking forward the drug strategy within establishments;
   (j) to provide effective training for staff in establishments on drug issues.
4. *To stifle the availability of illegal drugs on our streets*
   (a) to learn from and disseminate best practice around the Service;
   (b) to discriminate effectively between those prisoners whose activities cause most harm and those who genuinely wish to break their addiction;
   (c) to set targets for reduced availability of opiates and other drugs, and be vigilant for signs that prisoners may be switching from less to more damaging misuse;
   (d) to disrupt the distribution networks for illegal drugs in establishments;
   (e) to reward drug-free behaviour by providing incentives and earned privileges.

THE NATIONAL APPROACH

The Prison Service headquarters have now established a new Directorate of Regimes, which contains a drug strategy unit. This directorate has overall responsibility for implementing the new Prison Service drug strategy over the next decade and building on the solid framework established in the Drug Misuse in Prisons document. The Service has a key role to play in the Government's national strategy and supporting the UK Anti-Drugs Coordinator, by establishing effective partnerships with, amongst others, other agencies in the criminal justice system.

The policy of the Prison Service is not to tolerate any drug misuse in penal establishments. It has a responsibility to take appropriate steps to reduce the supply of and demand for illegal drugs, whilst reducing the opportunity for inmates to damage their health through abusing drugs. Effective intervention can result in significant harm reduction to individuals, their families and the communities they will be returning to on release.

The main priorities for the Prison Service are spelled out in 'Tackling Drugs in Prison' and are as follows:

* reducing recidivism amongst drug misusing offenders;
* increasing referrals for treatment;
* increasing treatment programme completions;
* deterring and detecting drug availability in prisons.

The Service intends to use the opportunity while inmates are in custody to make effective interventions and reduce significantly the damage caused to communities by offenders on release. This will be achieved by working closely with other statutory and non-statutory agencies and by carefully monitoring and evaluating performance.

The following specific measures are designed to ensure the strategy is successful:

(a) commissioning research into key aspects of the strategy;
(b) strengthening links between statutory and voluntary agencies;
(c) monitoring how funds are spent on drug testing and treatment programmes;
(d) concentrating on high-quality training on drug issues;
(e) maintaining a correct balance between security, health and regime issues;
(f) developing the scope of existing policy to include other substance abuse, notably alcohol abuse;
(g) improving its representation on Drug Action Teams locally.

This range of measures will be complemented by continuing action to reduce the supply of drugs in prisons by:

* searching prisoners and their visitors;
* making improvements to perimeter security;
* increasing the use of closed circuit television (CCTV);
* using active and passive drug dogs;
* taking action against visitors who are involved in drug-related offences at establishments.

DEVELOPING A LOCAL STRATEGY

The Governor has overall responsibility for developing the local drug strategy but he delegates responsibility for its effective implementation to the Drug Strategy Coordinator, who is a member of the Senior Management Group.

The Drug Strategy Coordinator is responsible for ensuring the following elements are incorporated into the local policy document:

- procedures that prevent drugs entering the establishment;
- arrangements for drug testing;
- forming and leading a multi-disciplinary team;
- assessing local needs and deciding priorities;
- devising an implementation plan which includes
  (a) performance measures,
  (b) monitoring arrangements,
  (c) regular reviews of the strategy;
- arrangements to identify prisoners with drug problems;
- the provision of counselling, support and a range of treatment programmes;
- participating in multi-agency partnerships which coordinate treatment, help and support to prisoners on discharge;
- staff training;
- liaison with the Area Drug Coordinator.

The local strategy is agreed with the Area Manager and incorporated into the Governor's business plan. It should concentrate attention on the following priorities:

- reducing the supply of and demand for drugs;
- reducing the health risks to staff, prisoners and the wider community which result from drug misuse;
- providing education classes and information about
  (a) the dangers of misusing drugs,
  (b) alternative ways to come off drugs,
  (c) how to reduce the risks of cross infection,
  (d) the availability of help.

Developing a multi-disciplinary team
The Drug Strategy Coordinator should lead a multi-disciplinary team with representatives from the following departments and external agencies:

- security department;
- prison discipline officers, including those based on the voluntary testing unit;
- probation team;
- health care centre or hospital;
- the education contractor;
- the chaplaincy team;
- the psychology department;
- the CARAT assessor or local contract manager;
- representatives from community-based agencies;
- the Board of Visitors (BoV).

The drug strategy team should meet regularly, normally quarterly, on a formal basis and circulate widely copies of the minutes of each meeting, including to the Area Drug Strategy Coordinator. The drug strategy team review the local policy document annually and monitor progress on the implementation plan by determining appropriate performance criteria to evaluate its effectiveness.

CONDUCTING A NEEDS ASSESSMENT LOCALLY

A clear picture of the local situation needs to be obtained before an effective strategy can be devised. There are five essential aspects to examine if the local needs assessment is to be comprehensive:

1. the extent of drug misuse;
2. the supply of drugs;
3. staff and prisoner understanding of drug misuse;
4. local arrangements to deal with drug problems;
5. the availability of resources to combat drug misuse.

The extent of drug misuse

Assessing the scale of the problem means collecting data which provides information about the level of drug misuse amongst the prisoner population. Potential sources of information are the following:

- the mandatory drug testing centre;
- health care screening reports;
- pre-sentence reports;
- intelligence contained in security information reports;
- surveys conducted with the prisoner population about their drug use which identify
  (a) any previous history of taking drugs,
  (b) the level of current usage,
  (c) how motivated prisoners are to tackle their drug problem,
  (d) reports on throughcare and discharge plans.

The supply of drugs

There are several sources of information about the supply of drugs in the prison, which include:

- measuring and analysing the level of drug finds in the establishment;
- intelligence obtained and collated by the security department;

- the result of searching visitors to the prison or Young Offender Institution (YOI);
- the number of visitors subject to a visits ban;
- drug finds when searching prisoners;
- the number of prisoners on closed visits;
- shared intelligence with the police liaison officer;
- intelligence obtained from prisoners;
- contact with community-based drug agencies.

Staff and prisoner understanding of drug misuse

The knowledge base of prison staff needs to be carefully assessed if staff training is to be targeted effectively. This should include training on blood-borne and communicable diseases, which includes the management of risk situations.

A comprehensive assessment needs to be made about the extent of prisoner understanding about the harmful effects of misusing drugs. They need to be aware of the health risks associated with sharing needles and the way viral infections such as hepatitis, and HIV, are transmitted.

These educational needs can be catered for by providing health education programmes and accredited drug awareness classes for prisoners.

Local arrangements to deal with drug problems

The local arrangements that currently exist in establishments to deal with drug misuse include:

- systematic random searching programmes;
- drug treatment programmes;
- the provision of information and education classes about drugs;
- counselling, assessment, referral, advice and throughcare services provided under the CARAT contract and rehabilitation services or therapeutic communities;
- self-help groups.

The availability of resources to combat drug misuse

Identifying the resources available to the establishment to tackle the drugs problem is a key task. This will include dedicated prison staff working on a voluntary testing unit or in the delivery of groups, non-prison-based staff from the Area Health Authority, probation officers, police liaison officers, community-based agencies, and staff made available to the establishment through the CARAT contract.

Identifying, collating and evaluating all this information enables a clear needs analysis to be made, and allows an action plan to be devised which can be achieved within a given timescale. One way to conduct this analysis and review the success of current strategies is to arrange an 'away day' at a local venue with the whole drug strategy team, including the Area Drug Coordinator where possible.

USING A MULTI-DISCIPLINARY APPROACH

Under the Comprehensive Spending Review (CSR), the Prison Service was allocated £76m to improve the availability and quality of drug treatment services to prisoners.

A key element of the Prison Service drug strategy are the Counselling, Assessment, Referral, Advice and Throughcare services (CARATs), which provide help to prisoners wishing to address their drug problems. It is particularly suitable for prisoners on remand or serving short sentences and who are not in custody long enough to benefit from a more intensive treatment such as a rehabilitation programme or therapeutic community.

Each Area Manager is responsible for ensuring every establishment in their area has a range of services which addresses the needs of those with low, moderate and severe drug problems.

The CARAT service is a fundamental part of the drug treatment strategy. Contracts were let in October 1999 to agencies able to work closely with prison and probation staff. CARAT services complement the existing sentence management process and provide an important link between:

- prisons and the courts, by providing information for bail applications and pre-sentence reports for those on remand;
- different establishments when prisoners are transferred, so that drug work commenced in one establishment can continue in another;
- different departments such as health care, probation and voluntary testing units;
- prisons and community-based agencies, to ensure there is continuity of care on release.

THE CARATS THROUGHCARE PROCESS

The CARAT service is a basic multi-disciplinary drug service which provides Counselling, Assessment, Referral, Advice/information and Throughcare for every prisoner who requests it. For anyone coming into prison for the first time this may be the only occasion they are offered help with their drug problems.

It is the starting point for assessing need and devising a treatment plan. This can lead to ongoing referrals to more intensive programmes if the sentence length makes this feasible. Appropriate treatment referrals are made and post-sentence support arranged, so effective aftercare can build on the benefits gained from prison-based treatment programmes.

The key priority is to link drug services in prisons with those in the community, ensuring that throughcare becomes a reality after release.

Accessing CARAT services

The aim of all CARAT services is to supply a method of identifying prisoners with drug problems, then provide an immediate and comprehensive response which is coordinated and systematic. The service is designed to be readily accessible and integrated with existing activities such as sentence management. Access to the CARAT service can be obtained at any of the seven stages shown in Figure 1, with referrals taking place as follows:

- self-referral;
- referral by a community-based agency which has previous involvement with the prisoner;
- referral by the family;
- through screening on reception by means of a risk or needs assessment;
- following a positive urine test result from voluntary or mandatory testing;
- by the security department after receiving a completed security information report (SIR);
- by a personal officer following a sentence management interview;
- by the probation department after making an assessment for home detention curfew, temporary release or a risk assessment;
- by education staff, the chaplaincy, workshop instructors and any member of staff who identifies a problem.

Assessing CARAT services

Many prisoners with a history of drug-related problems have not previously received help. Particular needs that have not traditionally been well catered for are those of women, young people, multiple drug users and those from different ethnic backgrounds. There are many drug misusers with undiagnosed and untreated mental health problems which CARAT services seek to identify and refer to other services for specialist treatment.

CARAT services are being evaluated by identifying the numbers of prisoners who receive treatment in custody, and who make contact with support services in the community on release.

The overall drug strategy will be judged by the extent to which reoffending levels reduce, and whether health improvements occur that can be attributable to a reduction in drug use.

MINIMUM STANDARDS

The CARAT system has seven inter-related stages which are illustrated in Figure 1:

1. Initial contact takes place normally on reception, but can be at any point in the sentence.
2. Referral to health care enables a clinical assessment and detoxification to take place.
3. A full assessment based on needs is undertaken.
4. The preparation of care plans supports the throughcare process and is reinforced by regular care reviews.

5. Counselling and groupwork address a prisoner's drug misuse problems.
6. Planning for release optimizes a prisoner's chances of managing the drug problem on release.
7. Post-release work establishes links with community-based agencies.

The agreed quality standards are clearly set out in the contracts for each of these seven stages. This enables a consistent and uniform service to be provided across the country, even when CARAT services are provided by a number of different suppliers.

Stage 1: Initial contact

On reception the prisoner is seen by either a specialist drug worker, a trained prison officer, a CARAT health care specialist or a probation officer. He is given advice and information about drugs and their effects; the hazards of sharing needles; the risk of overdosing and self-harm; the particular risks facing women drug users and the full range of services available in prison on release.

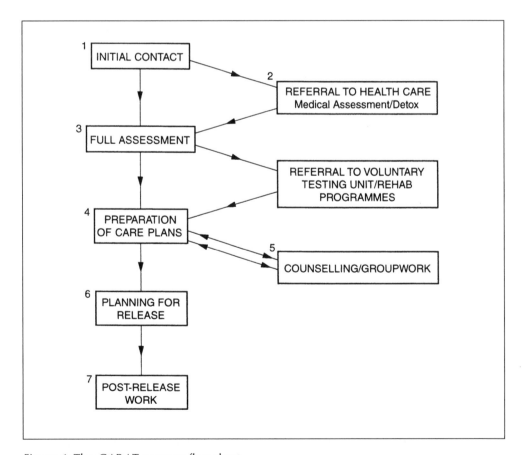

Figure 1: The CARAT process flowchart

At this stage data is collected on the numbers of prisoners provided with information, the scale of identifiable drug problems and those referred for the full CARAT assessment (Stage 3).

Stage 2: Referral to health care

On referral to health care, a CARAT-qualified health care worker makes a comprehensive assessment of the prisoners' physical and mental health. This involves obtaining further information from community health agencies and their GPs about the prisoners' medical history and prescribed medication. In appropriate cases, detoxification takes place.

Stage 3: Full assessment

During the following five working days, a comprehensive needs assessment is carried out by staff who are trained and have relevant experience of working with drug users. A standardized assessment process is used which covers the prisoners' history of drug use; the link between drug use and their offending behaviour; their need for services and treatment; and a list of recommendations.

The confidential nature of the service is explained to prisoners and their written consent obtained before external agencies, previously involved in their treatment, are contacted.

In the case of convicted prisoners, the CARAT assessor identifies whether further advice and guidance is appropriate, then makes referrals for CARAT support; detoxification; admission to a voluntary testing unit; an intensive rehabilitation programme and other services in the community.

Remand prisoners can request that their progress on detoxification or other treatment programmes is brought to the attention of:

- defence solicitors and the Crown Prosecution Service (CPS);
- bail information officers;
- probation staff compiling pre-sentence reports;
- community drug agencies, particularly when a community-based sentence is being considered.

The CARAT assessor will be concerned to establish whether a woman prisoner is pregnant, what child care arrangements she has made, and whether there is any likelihood that she may self-harm.

Following assessment, an initial care plan is agreed with the prisoner and produced by the CARAT assessor using a standard format.

Stage 4: Preparation of care plans

The purpose of the care plan is to agree a set of goals between the CARAT worker and the prisoner within a laid-down timescale. The care plan should be produced within ten working days and copies sent to the personal officer and other relevant depart-ments. Regular progress reviews with the prisoner are scheduled and the care plan is amended by mutual consent in the light of experience.

Stage 5: Counselling and groupwork

Ongoing services to the prisoner may take the form of one-to-one casework and be supplemented by individualized counselling or low-threshold groupwork. A number of groups may be offered, led by a facilitator or on a self-help basis. Counselling is provided to recognized standards and the models deployed are brief solution-focused therapy and motivational interviewing. Any counselling or groupwork provided is geared towards addressing goals set out in the care plan. Acupuncture and other complementary therapies may also be offered if considered appropriate.

Stage 6: Planning for release

Prior to discharge, a release plan is drawn up by the CARAT worker. The CARAT release plan, which should contribute to the overall sentence management release plan, includes an assessment of the prisoner's drug use prior to coming into prison and his response to treatment offered in custody. It sets out specific arrangements for post-release care, including an appointment with a named community drug worker to take place soon after release. Where the prisoner has been approved for release on Home Detention Curfew, the release plan is passed to the prison probation officer and the relevant community drug agency.

Stage 7: Post-release work

Seamless throughcare should be possible for prisoners who are discharged to a local address since the CARAT worker can provide support in the community for an initial period of up to eight weeks where community support from an agency cannot be arranged. Where the prisoner is being discharged to a distant address, it is likely to prove impractical for a community drugs worker from the relevant area to visit the prisoner before release. Liaison takes place between the prison and community, and the CARAT worker monitors arrangements and checks that the first post-release appointment is kept.

Drug Strategy Coordinator

The responsibility for managing the contract locally, and coordinating the work of those providing CARAT services with other disciplines within the establishment, lies with the Drug Strategy Coordinator, who is a member of the senior management team in each prison or Young Offender Institution.

CASE STUDY

John is assessed for CARAT services

Following sentence, John is interviewed on reception to prison and a needs assessment carried out when it becomes clear he has a drug-dependency problem. He is referred to the health care centre and seen by the medical officer and a CARAT health care specialist. Arrangements are made for him to receive detoxification treatment.

A comprehensive picture is built up about his previous drug use, with John's full cooperation, and contact is made with outside drug agencies and his GP, who provides the medical officer with information about his medical history and previous treatment. Following detoxification treatment, a full assessment is completed and arrangements made to admit John onto the voluntary testing unit. He signs a 'compact' which requires him to avoid using any drugs whilst on the VTU and to have regular voluntary tests.

A care plan is devised with his CARAT worker, which includes a number of goals to achieve within an agreed timescale. The care plan identifies a need for John to receive individual counselling, to attend a group and to receive post-release help in the form of supervision and aftercare by a community drug worker.

Following admission to the VTU, John commences individual counselling sessions and is soon accepted onto an accredited Enhanced Thinking Skills Course.

CHECKLIST

- Identify the four aims of 'Tackling Drugs in Prison' which link into the Government's national ten-year strategy.
- Describe the role of the Drug Strategy Unit based in headquarters.
- What are the main priorities of the Prison Service in relation to 'Tackling Drugs in Prison'?
- Who should be represented on the multi-disciplinary drug strategy team?
- What is the role of the Drug Strategy Coordinator?
- Which aspects of the local situation should be examined when conducting a comprehensive needs assessment?
- What is a Counselling, Assessment, Referral, Advice and Throughcare service?
- How can prisoners access CARAT services?
- Describe how the CARAT throughcare process works.
- What is the role of a CARAT assessor?
- When are care plans prepared on prisoners and by whom?
- What is the role of the Drug Strategy Coordinator?

CHAPTER 4

Drugs Prevention

REDUCING THE AVAILABILITY OF DRUGS

An important measure introduced in April 1999 supports the aim in the drug strategy to stifle the availability of illegal drugs in prisons, by taking firm and consistent action against all visitors and prisoners who smuggle drugs through visits. This applies to privately managed prisons as well as to directly managed prisons in the public sector.

Any visitor who attempts to smuggle drugs into a prison is liable to receive a ban of at least three months, followed by three months of closed visits. This applies to members of the family as well as friends. In addition to the general power to restrict or prevent entry to prisons (under Rules 34 and 35), the Prison Rules 1999 state in Rule 73 (YOI Rule 71A) that: 'The Secretary of State may, with a view to securing discipline and good order, or the prevention of crime, or in the interests of any persons, impose prohibitions on visits by a person to a prison, or to a prisoner ... for such periods of time as he considers necessary.'

Banning a visitor

The Governor is expected to impose a three month ban on visitors found smuggling drugs into the prison on visits. They are banned only under the following circumstances:

- if they are found in possession of drugs during a search;
- if they are seen during a visit passing an unauthorized item to a prisoner who is subsequently found in possession of the item at the end of the visit, or is unable to give a satisfactory explanation of what was passed;
- if the prisoner is found in possession of drugs at the end of the visit and it is established the drugs came in during the visit.

A visitor is not banned solely on the basis of a positive indication by a passive drug dog, although that may be sufficient grounds for conducting a search of the visitor.

The Governor can impose a longer ban than three months on a visitor if he considers it is appropriate, but he must review the ban every three months. Although the ban only applies to the prison where the incident occurred, Governors are encouraged to make sure the ban is re-imposed at the receiving prison for a similar period.

In exceptional circumstances the Governor can exercise his discretion and subject the visitor to a period of closed visits for a maximum period of six months. The Governor must consider carefully whether imposing a ban would cause disproportionate harm to the prisoner or visitor's rights, or infringe any rights protected under the European Convention of Human Rights. He must consider the following factors:

- the right of a prisoner or visitor to a family life (Article 8);
- the rights of children to have access to a parent (Article 9);
- the rights of a juvenile prisoner to have access to a parent;
- any exceptional compassionate reasons;
- where a ban would increase the risk of self-harm or suicide to the prisoner.

Governors continue to involve the police in all cases where a visitor is discovered smuggling drugs, and the police may decide to prosecute a visitor in addition to any administrative action the Governor takes.

Any visitor who is banned from visiting for a given period is informed in writing, and advised they have a right of appeal to the Governor. A standardized letter, used at most establishments, explains the reasons for the ban, its expiry date, that following the ban the visitor will be searched every visit and be obliged to take visits in closed conditions where no physical contact is possible.

Once the prisoner has been informed of the reason for the ban and the decision to impose closed visits, or any other restrictions, he can appeal using the normal request and complaint system.

Visitors strongly suspected of smuggling, but where no clear proof exists, are sent a warning letter pointing out the potential penalties of smuggling drugs into prisons. A warning notice to visitors (and prisoners) should be clearly displayed in every visits room and Visitor Centre. These notices explain the consequences of being caught smuggling drugs. These are:

- that visitors found smuggling drugs will be reported to the police;
- they are likely to be banned from the prison;
- the nature of closed visits;
- the visitors can expect to be searched every time they visit;
- the prisoner they visit is also likely to be disciplined;
- that if the visitor is being pressurized to bring drugs into prison, help is available.

Any visitor who is banned can, in exceptional circumstances, have the ban set aside temporarily by the Board of Visitors, in order to allow a visit to take place under Rule 35(6): 'The board of visitors may allow a prisoner an additional letter or visit in special circumstances, and may direct that a visit may extend beyond the normal duration.'

At the end of the ban and period of closed visits, visitors are then targeted for searches. This means they are given a full rub-down search every time they visit the prison and their property is thoroughly checked. The prisoner concerned is also given a rub down search, and possibly receives a full strip search, at the Governor's discretion.

Prisoners involved in smuggling drugs

Any prisoner thought to be involved in smuggling drugs through visits can be dealt with through the disciplinary system or placed on closed visits. It is not necessary for there to be prima facie evidence to place a prisoner on closed visits; intelligence obtained from a letter or telephone call may be sufficient. Being observed receiving something from a visitor, then when challenged being unable to retrieve the object in question or give a satisfactory explanation, is sufficient evidence to assume an involvement in drug smuggling, and grounds for taking any of the following action:

- placing prisoners on closed visits for a specific period
    (a) remand prisoners for three months,
    (b) convicted prisoners for the equivalent of three months' statutory and earned privilege visits;
- targeting for searches;
- referring for drug counselling;
- reviewing their status on the Incentive and Earned Privilege Scheme (IEPS);
- reviewing their continuance on a voluntary testing unit;
- reviewing their allocation;
- reviewing their suitability for Home Detention Curfew;
- giving a mandatory drug test on reasonable suspicion;
- following at least one finding of guilt on adjudication for drug smuggling, placing them on the frequent drug-testing programme.

Resisting coercion

Some prisoners put pressure on their visitors and other prisoners to bring drugs into the establishment on their behalf. Staff are aware of this practice and are on the lookout for signs of bullying and coercion. This can be countered in a number of ways, including the following:

- making visitors aware of the consequences of drug smuggling by making leaflets available and displaying posters in the Visitor Centre;
- providing a drugs amnesty bin where drugs can be deposited before visitors enter the visits room;
- having a confidential telephone line for visitors to disclose they are under pressure;
- having an approachable member of staff available to offer advice and gather intelligence;
- establishing good links with the local police and sharing intelligence.

NOTICE TO VISITORS
Measures To Tackle Drug Smuggling Through Visits

It is an offence to bring drugs into prison. If you are found to have brought drugs into the prison or handed them over to a prisoner, we will call the police, and we will press for charges of possession with intent to supply. This can result in a prison sentence.

Since April 1999, additional measures apply.

If you are found in possession of drugs, or if you are caught passing drugs to a prisoner, you will be liable to the following:

*   To be banned from the prison. You will normally be banned for at least three months. This means you will not be able to visit any prisoner here. If the prisoner you were visiting moves, the ban will normally follow to the new prison.
*   After the ban, to have your visits in closed or non-contact conditions. This will normally be for a further three months. This means you will not be able to touch the prisoner and there may be a glass screen between you.
*   To be searched every time you visit until we are satisfied you are no longer a risk.

Whether to ban you or impose closed visits, and for how long, are matters for the Governor. You can appeal against the decision by writing to or telephoning the Governor.

You should also be aware that prisoners found to be involved in smuggling drugs through visits are treated very firmly. Drug smuggling can result in disciplinary proceedings, which carry a wide range of penalties, including up to 42 additional days to be served in prison. It can also result in closed visits, additional urine tests, extra searches (which may be strip searches), and it can affect what privileges they are allowed, their security category, and what prison they are sent to next.

Please do not put your friend or loved one in this position by agreeing to requests for drugs, and never bring drugs as a present.

If you or your prisoner are being pressurized to bring drugs in, you can speak in confidence to staff at the Visitor Centre.

Governor

Figure 2: Notice to visitors document

TACKLING THE SUPPLY OF DRUGS

A crucial task is to make it increasingly difficult for drugs to find a route into prisons in the first place. The task is huge as drugs are easy to conceal and the rewards for success are immense. The legal position is clearly set out in The Prison Rules (Rule 70) 1999: 'No person shall throw into or deposit in a prison ... or convey to a prisoner, or deposit in any place with intent that it shall come into the possession of a prisoner, ... any controlled drug.' Whilst part of this strategy is aimed at deterring people from attempting to bring drugs into prison, a number of measures can be taken which increase the likelihood of detection, and so reduce the amount of drugs getting into circulation.

It is unrealistic to expect the supply of drugs into prisons to be completely eliminated. Mr Keith Hellawell, the UK Anti-Drugs Coordinator, highlighted the difficulties when he gave evidence to the Home Affairs Committee on Drugs and Prisons on 30 March 1999:

> They could introduce a totalitarian regime where there were no open visits with friends and family, where everyone who worked in the prison and everyone who delivered to the prison and everyone who provided a service for the prison would be screened and tested upon every occasion they entered the prison. I think that would be unacceptable in a democratic society ... it is the balance we have to achieve.

Measures which can be taken include the following:

- improving perimeter security and searching;
- supervising visits effectively;
- using CCTV;
- intelligence-gathering and the use of informants;
- controlling the use of prescribed drugs;
- mandatory drug testing.

Security and searching

Prison Rule 71 states that 'Any person or vehicle entering or leaving a prison may be stopped, examined and searched.' Searching programmes should be proactive rather than purely routine, and kept up-to-date and conducted efficiently. Searching should be carried out on a random cycle, which means it is completely unpredictable to prisoners. The prison staff need to be well-trained and supervised by local managers to ensure a consistent standard of searching is carried out. Using specialist dog-searching teams on an occasional basis is valuable in flushing out drugs, particularly in establishments which do not have their own dog section.

The perimeter security can be improved by floodlighting the wall and extending CCTV coverage to ensure there is comprehensive coverage, with no blind spots. Electronic detection devices can be installed, and dogs used to patrol the sterile area in higher security establishments (where the cost can be justified) on the grounds that these prisoners must be held in very secure conditions with a high priority given at all times to holding them securely in custody.

Security can be improved in most establishments by increasing the frequency of fence patrols and searching the ground adjacent to the perimeter fence, before prisoners are allowed to leave the wings to take part in work or other activities. This allows any illicit items thrown over the wall or perimeter fence to be retrieved. It is a common occurrence in lower security prisons for drugs to be placed inside an object which is thrown over the fence for retrieval later by a prisoner. The interception by staff before prisoners gain access to these objects is a powerful deterrent.

Supervising visits effectively

The visits area is a particularly vulnerable place for drugs to enter prisons. Although some visitors are not deterred by the measures outlined to deal with drug smuggling, the development of good liaison arrangements with the local police has proved an effective strategy.

Reviewing the quality of the systems to supervise prisoners and their visitors effectively in the visits area has led to changes in visiting procedures. Altering the route visitors take at some establishments had ensured that they cannot become contaminated after searching procedures. Increasing the level of supervision by re-positioning staff in strategic positions, and ensuring visitors who have to visit the toilet during a visit receive a further search, has also proved beneficial. Redesigning visits furniture, so that special low-level tables and fixed chairs are used, makes it more difficult to pass unauthorized articles and drugs. This measure coupled to the use of closed circuit television (CCTV) is particularly effective.

Using CCTV

CCTV has a much wider application than purely being deployed in visits areas; its use has contributed to perimeter security and helped detect objects thrown over the prison wall or perimeter fence. It is also used in living accommodation units, in the gate area and is positioned strategically in the car park to good effect.

Most establishments are introducing CCTV in the visits area where it is proving to be an effective weapon against drugs. It is being given a high priority in all visits areas, despite the high cost of installation which can be as much as £50k per establishment. CCTV is now (at March 2000) in the visits area of 118 establishments, together with low-level and fixed furniture. CCTV can be staff intensive, as the ideal set-up involves the monitoring of live recordings. However, it is an effective way to gather evidence of drug smuggling which is used in adjudications or given to the police to assist them in criminal proceedings.

Intelligence-gathering

Targeting visitors suspected by the police and prison authorities of trafficking can be carried out effectively using systems for gathering and collating information

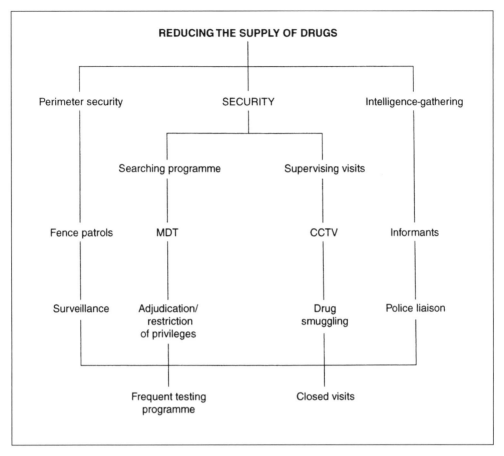

Figure 3: Reducing the supply of drugs flowchart

which have been developed jointly. Intelligence is shared with customs and the police as part of the strategy to reduce the supply of drugs entering establishments. As a consequence, searching strategies are being refined and suspects targeted efficiently.

Effective police liaison arrangements mean the police respond promptly to requests to search visitors suspected of smuggling drugs. Some prison staff in establishments are receiving joint training with the police, so suspects can be detained and evidence preserved correctly. The number of visitors being arrested for drug-related offences is currently running at over a thousand per annum. Where the courts are using exemplary sentences, this is acting as a big deterrent.

The use of informants in prison is being developed and this helps in the intelligence-gathering process. Monitoring correspondence and tape recording tele-phone conversations provides invaluable information, whilst examining for trends in a prisoner's spending habits and private cash transactions can be revealing. Regular transactions to certain addresses are often a sign of drug dealing.

Controlling the use of prescribed drugs

Care has to be exercised in dispensing medicines such as methadone as there is a ready market amongst the prisoner population for all kinds of prescribed drugs. Methadone must be prepared in a liquid form and care exercised when it is administered to prisoners. The prisoner is observed by the nurse or health care worker while he swallows the drug in the health care centre or hospital. To avoid any possibility of mistaken identity or some other subterfuge occurring, each prescription has a photograph of the prisoner attached to it.

DRUG TESTING

The use of mandatory drug testing is proving to be an effective strategy to detect drug misuse. HM Prison Service Annual Report and Accounts 1998–1999 states that the in-year target set for random drug testing was: 'To ensure that the rate of positive random testing for drugs is lower than 20%' (Key Performance Indicator 3). The rate of positive tests was exceeded as the overall rate of positive tests was 18.6 per cent, which is the lowest level since testing began.

An improved target for 1999–2000 was set: 'To ensure that the rate of positive results from random tests is lower than 18.5%'. This target was easily achieved; the latest figures are included in the Annual Report 1999–2000, published by HMSO on 24 July 2000, and are 14.2% of random mandatory tests proved positive.

Drug-testing performance

The rate of positive testing varies considerably throughout establishments and this needs to be addressed. The margin between the best and worst performers is significant, as the following figures taken from the statistical information tables in the Annual Report 1998–9 clearly demonstrate:

Drug Testing: Female Establishments
Female local prisons
Best performer: New Hall   4.8%
Worst performer: Eastwood Park   15.3%

Female closed prisons
Best performer: Cookham Wood   5.9%
Worst performer: Send   19.6%

Female open prisons
Best performer: East Sutton Park   4.2%
Worst performer: Drake Hall   17.7%

Drug Testing: Male Establishments
Male local prisons

Best performer:	Haslar	2.4%
Worst performer:	Parc	44.6%

Dispersal prisons

Best performer:	Wakefield	1.2%
Worst performer:	Frankland	17.7%

Category B prisons

Best performer:	Albany	1.3%
Worst performer:	Lowdham Grange	30.7%

Category C prisons

Best performer:	Blantyre House	0.7%
Worst performer:	Featherstone	41.9%

Category D male open prisons

Best performer:	Morton Hall	8.2%
Worst performer:	Hollesley Bay	25.6%

Drug Testing: Young Offender Institutions
Male closed Young Offender Institutions

Best performer:	Onley	3.9%
Worst performer:	Guys Marsh	33.9%

Male open Young Offender Institutions

Best performer:	Hatfield	15.7%
Worst performer:	Thorn Cross	23.1%

The revised strategy

The strategy was revised in 1999 to provide a mix of random and targeted mandatory drug testing in establishments based on research evidence which showed that targeted mandatory testing was having a deterrent effect. This revised approach means that small establishments of fewer than 400 prisoners are required to random test a minimum of 10 per cent of the population each month, but not to exceed a maximum of 15 per cent of the population.

Larger establishments (over 400 prisoners) can reduce the random testing target to a minimum of 5 per cent, and they too must not exceed 15 per cent. However, targeted testing is to be stepped up commensurately so that the overall level of mandatory drug testing is not decreased. Targeted testing is to concentrate on new receptions, on suspicion, risk assessments and on those being tested under the frequent testing programme. The aim is to test at least 10 per cent of the prisoner population each month from September 1999.

Year	Total	Cannabis	Opiates/heroin	Cocaine
1996–7	24.4%	19.95%	5.4%	0.2%
1997–8	20.8%	16.5%	4.2%	0.2%
1998–9	18.3%	14.0%	4.4%	0.3%
1999–2000	14.2%	10.3%	4.4%	0.2%

Figure 4: Positive random test results chart

A further change introduced in August 1999 is for 14 per cent of random and targeted testing to take place at weekends, with testing taking place at all establishments at least every three weeks. This addresses the reported problem that prisoners were having drug holidays at the weekends whereby they could take hard drugs in the knowledge that they would be highly unlikely to test positive after the weekend.

PASSIVE AND ACTIVE DRUG DETECTION DOGS

An integral part of the strategy to restrict the supply of drugs into establishments is the use of passive and active drug detection dogs. In dispersal prisons and establishments holding category A inmates, the use of patrol dogs is routine and drug detection dogs are regularly deployed. Although it is not obligatory for other establishments to have dogs, the Prison Service drugs strategy has encouraged their widespread use, including in low security establishments. The main improvements have been 60 new passive dogs, 12 new active dogs and 39 additional handlers in 1999/2000.

Passive Drug Detection dogs (PDD dogs) work only whilst on a collar and lead and under the direct control of a qualified dog handler. Their role is to search for drugs on visitors and inmates and to screen staff. They are capable of detecting and passively alerting their handler to the presence of drug-taking equipment and the drugs amphetamine sulphates, cannabis, cocaine, crack and heroin.

The dogs have the appropriate temperament to avoid reacting to any provocation they encounter. They can work comfortably on their own or as part of a dog team.

Active Drug Detection Dogs (ADD dogs) are used to search for the same wide range of drugs and drug-related equipment anywhere in the establishment. They are used to carry out routine searches and to check that buildings, such as living units or workshops, are drug-free. They can work off the lead providing they are always under the control of a qualified handler, and can be used singly or as part of a dog team. ADD dogs must be able to remain composed, not to react to any provocation and to cope with noisy and adverse working conditions, including night work.

These dogs are not used to search people, but can act as a visible deterrent in areas such as the gate and in the visits room.

Operational standards

Once appointed, dog handlers complete an initial training programme which leads to an accredited certificate of qualification. Handlers have to possess personal skills and specialized technical knowledge, which includes being well versed in the relevant health and safety procedures.

Deploying an ADD dog safely means being able to demonstrate evidence of the following competencies:

* basic dog handling skills;
* caring for the dog properly;
* exercising full control over the dog in all operating conditions;
* understanding canine behaviour;
* a close rapport with their dog.

Specialist drug detection dogs attend an annual development course which consists of a minimum of 40 hours' continuation training. All dogs are assessed on an annual basis by accredited assessors and a certificate of accreditation, valid for twelve months, is issued to those who achieve the standard. Those dogs that fail the assessment process are removed from operational duties and, if they are unable to meet the required standard within three months, can be removed from service altogether.

The quality standards that apply to the care and deployment of drug dogs include:

* keeping detailed records of all searches undertaken by the dogs;
* maintaining dog training records, pedigree details, veterinary records of illnesses, accidents and treatment received, and micro-chipping details;
* the feeding and dietary requirements of each dog;
* the facilities within the establishment for the care of the dog and its equipment, including the stand-down kennels;
* the kennel facilities at the handler's home;
* accurately accounting for all drug-training aids, ensuring samples are replaced annually and safely disposed of.

It is a requirement that all dog handlers have clear lines of responsibility and accountability, and that dogs are always deployed safely.

CASE STUDY

John is involved in smuggling drugs through visits

John's common-law wife attracts the attention of the passive drug dog while waiting to enter the visits room. The visit is allowed to proceed but the couple are kept under surveillance by the CCTV cameras.

During the social visit, she is observed passing a small package to John who surreptitiously secretes the package about his person. The whole incident is recorded on CCTV and prison staff supervising visits are alerted to the incident by radio; they swoop on John and his visitor. The visit is terminated and his visitor is taken away and arrested by the local police. John is given a strip search and subsequently charged under Prison Rule 51 Paragraph 24 with 'receiving any controlled drug, during the course of a visit', which is the new offence introduced in The Prison Rules 1999 to deal with drug smuggling and bringing unauthorized items to social visits.

The Governor decides to use his powers under Prison Rule 73, in line with the displayed Notice to Visitors, and imposes a ban of three months followed by three months of closed visits. However, John decides to appeal using the request and complaints system, on the grounds that this would prevent him seeing his children and contravene his rights under the European Convention of Human Rights (Article 7). After consulting the prison-based probation service, the Governor decides on compassionate grounds to amend his original decision and places John on three months of closed visits.

CHECKLIST

- In what circumstances might a Governor decide to ban a visitor?
- What is the normal ban imposed on a visitor found smuggling drugs?
- How does a Governor assess whether imposing a ban would cause disproportionate harm?
- Under what circumstances can the Board of Visitors temporarily set aside a Governor's ban on a visitor?
- What are the main reasons prisoners put pressure on their families to bring in drugs?
- How can the coercion of visitors be countered?
- What are closed visits?
- Identify measures that could make drug smuggling more difficult.
- Would the introduction of a totalitarian regime eliminate the problem of drugs coming into prisons?
- How are the arrangements for mandatory drug testing being altered to make it more effective?
- Define the role of a Passive Drug Detection Dog.
- How are Active Drug Detection Dogs used in establishments?
- What quality standards are applicable to dog handlers?
- Why are drug dogs assessed on an annual basis?

CHAPTER 5

Mandatory Drug Testing

THE LEGAL PROVISIONS

The Prison Rules 1999 came into effect on 1 April 1999. They set out clearly the purpose of imprisonment: 'The purpose of the training and treatment of convicted prisoners shall be to encourage them to lead a good and useful life' (Rule 3). They highlight the importance of keeping outside contacts, encouraging family links, including visits, and working towards preparing for their release:

> Special attention shall be paid to the maintenance of such relationships between a prisoner and his family as are desirable in the best interests of both. A prisoner shall be encouraged and assisted to establish and maintain such relations with persons and agencies outside prison as may, in the opinion of the governor, best promote the interests of his family and his own social rehabilitation. (Rules 4 and 5)

The emphasis is on sentence management and a throughcare approach that pays close attention to helping the prisoner successfully re-integrate into society on release, and avoid reoffending: 'From the beginning of a prisoner's sentence, consideration shall be given, in consultation with the appropriate after-care organisation, to the prisoner's future and the assistance to be given him on or after his release.'

Offences against discipline

The Prison Rules 1999 and the YOI (Amendment) (No. 2) Rules 1999 mean that young offenders must be charged under YOI Rule 50, and adults are charged under Rule 51. Charges under Rule 51 are laid against adult prisoners or remand prisoners irrespective of their age and whether unconvicted or unsentenced.

There are two specific charges which relate to controlled drugs, paragraphs 9 and 24, but several charges relate to activity associated with illicit drug taking. The full list of offences against discipline is as follows:

1. *Commits any assault*
   This applies to any unlawful use of force against another person. The adjudicator

will consider the seriousness of any injuries sustained as this is an important factor when deciding whether to involve the police. The victim also has the right to make a formal complaint to the police if a criminal offence has been committed. Normally, if the offence would warrant a charge of grievous bodily harm being brought in the community, then the police become involved and a prosecution may result. An assault charge makes no distinction between assaults against staff or other prisoners, although any assault against a member of staff is considered very serious.

2. *Detains any person against his will*
   This charge is laid against a hostage-taker. Such an offence is always formally referred to the police for criminal proceedings to be initiated.

3. *Denies access to any part of the prison to any officer (other than a prisoner) who is at the prison for the purpose of working there*
   This charge covers instances where barricades occur, but may also be used if an inmate prevents an officer intervening to break up a fight.

4. *Fights with any person*
   A fight is a mutual assault. It occurs when there is an exchange of blows or when both inmates wrestle with each other. Some fights turn out on further investigation to be assaults, particularly if one of the inmates involved is able to demonstrate they were acting in self-defence.

5. *Intentionally endangers the health or personal safety of others or, by his conduct, is reckless whether such health or safety is endangered*
   A common example of this offence is when an inmate tampers with the mains supply in order to wire up a radio or some other electrical item.

6. *Intentionally obstructs an officer in the execution of his duty, or any person (other than a prisoner) who is at the prison for the purpose of working there, in the performance of his work*
   This normally means causing a physical obstruction, but can also apply if an inmate deliberately provides false information to an officer.

7. *Escapes or absconds from prison or from legal custody*
   The definition of an escape is when a physical obstacle has to be overcome such as the perimeter wall or fence. Absconds occur when inmates in open conditions abuse trust by going off limits, or fail to return to the establishment by an agreed time.

8. *Fails to comply with any condition upon which he is temporarily released under Rule 9*
   This relates to the specific conditions included on the licence issued to cover a period of temporary release. A prisoner can only be released
   (a) on compassionate grounds or for the purpose of receiving medical treatment,
   (b) to engage in employment or voluntary work,
   (c) to receive instruction or training which cannot reasonably be provided in the prison,
   (d) to enable him to participate in any proceedings before any court, tribunal or inquiry,
   (e) to enable him to consult with his legal adviser in circumstances where it is not reasonably practical for the consultation to take place in the prison,

   (f)   to assist any police officer in any enquiries,
   (g)   to facilitate the prisoner's transfer between prisons,
   (h)   to assist him in maintaining family ties or in his transition from prison life to freedom,
   (i)   to enable him to make a visit in the locality of the prison, as a privilege as part of the published Incentive and Earned Privilege Scheme in the establishment.
9. *Administers a controlled drug to himself or fails to prevent the administration of a controlled drug to him by another person*
   A controlled drug as defined in The Prison Rules 1999 (Rule 2) means any drug which is a controlled drug for the purpose of the Misuse of Drugs Act 1971(2).
10. *Is intoxicated as a consequence of knowingly consuming any alcoholic beverage*
   This is the more serious of two alcohol-related charges and applies if the behaviour exhibited is consistent with intoxication.
11. *Knowingly consumes any alcoholic beverage other than that provided to him pursuant to a written order under rule 25(1)*
   This is the less serious alcohol-related charge and relates to the consumption of alcohol which has not been prescribed. The exception allowed for under Rule 25(1) is where a medical practitioner, who is a fully registered person within the meaning of the Medical Act 1983(7), makes a written order specifying the amount of intoxicating liquor that has been prescribed to a named prisoner.
12. *Has in his possession:*
   (a)   any unauthorized article, or
   (b)   a greater quantity of any article than he is authorized to have
      (a)   This applies to an item an inmate has in possession that does not appear on the privilege list.
      (b)   Often used when an inmate is suspected of engaging in illegal trading or baroning-type activities, and is associated with bullying.
13. *Sells or delivers to any person any unauthorized article*
   This covers supplying drugs or the illicit trading of items that are not permitted in possession.
14. *Sells or, without permission, delivers to any person any article which he is allowed to have only for his own use*
   This charge applies if another inmate lends out their personal radio or other permitted item. This is often associated with bullying and linked to the drug-taking culture, in the experience of staff.
15. *Takes improperly any article belonging to another person or to a prison*
   This charge is the equivalent to a charge of theft.
16. *Intentionally or recklessly sets fire to any part of a prison or any other property, whether or not his own*
   This applies to instances of arson.
17. *Destroys or damages any part of a prison or any other property, other than his own*
   This covers 'cell smash-ups', any damage to prison property, or intentional damage inflicted on another inmate's property.
18. *Absents himself from any place he is required to be or is present at any place where he is not authorized to be*

Inmates who wander are generally assumed to be up to no good. One known motive is to drop off drugs and other illicit substances for other inmates to collect later.

19. *Is disrespectful to any officer, or any person (other than a prisoner) who is at the prison for the purpose of working there, or any person visiting a prison*
   Inmates who are rude to auxiliary staff, civilians, Officer Support Grades (OSGs), official visitors or the relatives of other prisoners are committing a disciplinary offence.

20. *Uses threatening, abusive or insulting words or behaviour*
   This charge is used when inmates lose their temper, use bad language, or become abusive towards staff.

21. *Intentionally fails to work properly or, being required to work, refuses to do so*
   This applies to any convicted inmate who refuses to work, or attend educational classes, and is medically fit to carry out the required duties.

22. *Disobeys any lawful order*
   It is not necessary for a member of staff to preface any instruction by the words 'I am giving you a direct order ...' as some inmates mistakenly believe. Any polite request to carry out or refrain from doing something constitutes an order, providing it is reasonable and lawful.

23. *Disobeys or fails to comply with any rule or regulation applying to him*
   The rule or regulation can be a local rule that only applies to a particular establishment. Providing steps have been taken to inform inmates of the particular requirements, they are obliged to comply with them.

24. *Receives any controlled drug, or, without the consent of an officer, any other article, during the course of a visit (not being an interview such as is mentioned in Rule 38)*
   This is a new offence to deal with the smuggling of drugs and other unauthorized items through social visits but does not cover legal visits. Rule 38 (or YOI Rule 50 paragraph 22) refers to visits by a legal adviser to a prisoner who is involved in any civil or criminal proceedings.

Since August 2000, four new offences came into force:

   1A   Commits any racially aggravated assault;
   17A Causes racially aggravated damage to any part of a prison (or young offenders institution) or any other property other than his own;
   20A Uses threatening, abusive or insulting racist words or behaviour;
   24A Displays, attaches to or draws on any part of a prison threatening, abusive or insulting racist words, drawings, symbols or other material.

COMPULSORY TESTING FOR CONTROLLED DRUGS

The Criminal Justice and Public Order Act 1994 amended the Prison Act 1952(11) by adding section 16A. Under this section, subject to there being an authorization in force for the prison, a prison officer has the power to request a prisoner to provide a sample of urine for testing: 'The Prison Rules 1999 requires a prisoner to provide a sample of urine for the purpose of ascertaining whether he has any controlled drugs in his body' (Rule 50). There are a number of conditions that have to be satisfied under these rules and these are as follows:

- an officer shall ... inform the prisoner that he is required to provide a sample in accordance with 16A of the Prison Act 1952, and that a refusal to provide a sample may lead to disciplinary proceedings being brought against him (section 3);
- the prisoner is required to provide a fresh sample free from any adulteration (section 4);
- the officer shall make such arrangements and give the prisoner such instructions ... in order to prevent or detect its adulteration or falsification (section 5);
- the prisoner required to give the sample may be kept apart from other prisoners for a period not exceeding one hour whilst the necessary arrangements are made (section 6);
- a prisoner who is unable to provide a sample of urine when required to do so may be kept apart from other prisoners until he has provided the required sample ... for a period of not more than 5 hours (section 7);
- the prisoner providing the sample shall be afforded ... privacy for the purposes of providing the sample as may be consistent with the need to prevent or detect adulteration or falsification of the sample, in particular shall not be required to provide such a sample in the sight of the opposite sex (section 8).

Inmates are required to provide a urine sample for the purpose of drug testing under the following circumstances:

- *Risk assessment*
  Anyone being considered for a position of trust on an outside work party, or for release on temporary licence.
- *On reception*
  Whenever inmates return from a period of release on temporary licence, on first admission or on transfer to the establishment. Disciplinary action is not taken against anyone on first reception if the drug detected has a minimum waiting period which exceeds the length of time in custody and, as such, it cannot be clearly established that the drug misuse took place in prison.
- *On reasonable suspicion*
  If prison staff have reasonable grounds to suspect someone is taking drugs.
- *The frequent test programme*
  Anyone found guilty of misusing drugs in custody on more than one occasion can be placed on the frequent testing programme and expected to provide a sample on a regular basis. A programme of mandatory frequent testing has been introduced for all prisoners who test positive for class A drugs.
- *Random testing*
  An inmate's name may be selected on a totally random basis by computer for drug testing. Each month a proportion (5% or 10%) of the total population are tested in this way. Establishments are required to undertake 14% of mandatory drug tests.

Once an inmate has been selected for drug testing, he is taken to the drug-testing centre and required to provide a urine sample; he is given a maximum of five hours to produce a sample. This sample is sent away to a laboratory for analysis together with full details of any medication prescribed to the inmate, subject to the prisoner giving their consent to disclose medical information.

Refusal to provide a sample within the time limit means that the inmate is disobeying a lawful order. This results in a disciplinary charge under Rule 51 paragraph 22.

The length of time that drugs remain in the body varies, depending on the drug taken, the frequency of use and the individual's metabolism. The following are the minimum waiting periods before an inmate may be charged after first reception into prison, or charged again with a further offence:

Amphetamines including methamphetamines	4 days
Barbiturates, except phenobarbital	5 days
Phenobarbital	30 days
Benzodiazepines	30 days
Cannabis, light or moderate use (once or twice a week)	10 days
heavy to chronic use (daily)	30 days
Cocaine	4 days
Methadone	5 days
LSD	3 days
Opiates including morphine and codeine	7 days

These time periods represent the minimum waiting periods before a charge can safely be laid after first reception into custody. They are also the minimum period between samples that must elapse before disciplinary action for the same drug can take place.

The Mandatory Drug Test Authorization Form

Inmates required to give a urine sample are handed a Mandatory Drug Test Authorization Form. This sets out the reasons for requesting a sample and explains the procedure – how the sample is split at the point of collection into separate containers which are sealed in the inmate's presence; how inmates who wish to dispute any positive result can arrange for an independent analysis to take place at their own expense, within a period of twelve months; and their liability to be placed on report if they fail to cooperate or if they provide a positive sample.

The form contains a consent to medical disclosure which asks the inmate to sign one of the following statements:

- During the past 30 days I have not used any medication issued to me by Health Care.
- During the past 30 days I have used medicine issued to me by Health Care. I understand that some medication issued by Health Care may affect the result of the test. I give my consent to the Medical Officer to provide details of this treatment to the prison authorities.

The Prison Service Chain of Custody procedure

A copy of this is handed to each person being tested. It sets out the seventeen-point procedure which must be followed precisely if the tests are to be valid.

The inmate is asked to make a declaration in the following terms:

1. I understand why I was required to provide the sample and what may happen if I fail to comply with this requirement.
2. The urine sample I have given was my own and freshly provided.
3. The sample was divided into two bottles and sealed in my presence with seals initialled and dated by me.
4. The seals used on these bottles carry a barcode identical to the barcode attached to this form.

Once the sample has been collected it is divided into two tubes, sealed with tamper-proof seals, then placed in a chain of custody bag in the inmate's presence. It is not opened until it arrives at the laboratory.

At the laboratory, the sample tubes and seals are checked to make sure they have not been damaged or tampered with, the barcodes on the seals are checked with each other and the barcode label on the chain of custody form, which the inmate signed. Any discrepancies or signs of damage result in the sample being rejected for testing by the laboratory.

TESTING POSITIVE

There are three types of tests that are carried out in the mandatory drug testing (MDT) process: an initial *screening test*, the *confirmation test* and an *independent analysis*.

The Screening Test

All urine samples are subject to an initial screening test which uses a process known as *immunoassay* to identify samples which contain no drugs at all. The screening test is very effective at identifying samples testing negative but not so reliable at indicating that definite drug misuse has occurred.

Once the test results have been returned to the establishment and the effect of any prescribed medication assessed (providing consent has been given for medical disclosure), the inmate is informed.

If the result is positive, the inmate is charged under Rule 51 paragraph 9. If, at the disciplinary hearing, the inmate enters a plea of not guilty, the hearing will be adjourned to allow for a more sophisticated confirmation test to be made.

The Confirmation Test

The confirmation test has a high level of accuracy and reliability. It is a sophisticated two-stage process known as *Gas Chromatography/Mass Spectrometry (GC/MS)* and is capable of identifying the precise nature of any drug contained in the sample, and distinguishing between drug misuse and prescribed medication.

The accuracy of the confirmation test can be gauged from evidence available from 1997 of samples screening positive that were sent for confirmation test:

- 82.7 per cent of samples that screened positive were confirmed as positive (6838 samples out of a total of 8268).
- 94.5 per cent of those samples that screened positive for cannabis were confirmed as positive.
- Until 1999, no independent analysis had come up with a different result to the confirmation test result. In this unusual case the urine in the 'B' tube did not seem to be the same as that in the 'A' tube.

The Confirmation Test Report

The report is similar in format to the screening report and contains the establishment barcode and the sample collection date. It includes the results of all confirmation tests, both negative and positive, which are expressed in the following language:

- *Negative consistent with prescribed medicine*
  A positive test result which is consistent with taking prescribed medication from the health centre.
- *Positive, not consistent with prescribed medication listed*
  A statement which means the prescribed medication does not contain the drug found in the urine sample tested.
- *Opiates: positive, consistent with abuse of heroin*
  The substance 6-monoacetylmorphine (6-MAM) is only found in heroin, so the laboratory can be certain heroin is present in a urine sample when 6-MAM is detected.

Some drugs are contained in prescribed medication – codeine is found in some painkillers and migraine tablets and can give a positive test for opiates. Other prescribed drugs that give a positive result include tranquillizers and methadone, which is used for detoxing heroin addicts. A positive result for cannabis, however, cannot be caused by prescribed medication.

Once the results of the confirmation test are known, the disciplinary hearing can resume.

Independent laboratory analysis

A sample can be sent to an independent laboratory if inmates remain convinced that a positive test result is wrong. It is their responsibility to arrange this and pay the appropriate laboratory fee, normally at least £100, which may be met from Legal Aid.

Once a request for an independent analysis has been made the adjudication has to be adjourned to allow the necessary arrangements to be made. The original sample was divided equally into two tubes and labelled A and B. The B sample is stored securely in a freezer at the laboratory used by the Prison Service, where it is retained until the inmate or his legal adviser has found a laboratory prepared to conduct the independent analysis. A list of laboratories is kept in each establishment and can be obtained from MDT staff.

The procedure to release the sample for independent analysis is that the inmate or legal adviser provides the adjudicator with evidence of intent to arrange an independent analysis and asks them to authorize the release of the B sample and send it to the laboratory of their choice. A timescale of approximately 6 weeks is given in which prisoners and solicitors must ensure the arrangements for completion of an independent analysis of a positive MDT sample.

Once the independent analysis has been conducted, the report will be sent to the inmate or legal adviser. This report can be used as evidence, providing the adjudicating Governor is allowed to read the whole report.

The Prison Service has made it clear that it will not tolerate the use of drugs in prison and will do everything possible to reduce the availability and demand for drugs. Although it intends to try to educate, advise and treat anyone who has a drug problem, it also has a clear duty to bring disciplinary proceedings against drug abusers.

QUALITY CONTROL

The Blind Performance Challenge Programme

The laboratory is audited by the Prison Service who have their own quality assurance scheme, the Blind Performance Challenge Programme, which operates in the following way.

At regular intervals, Tackler Analytical (a drug standards company) sends samples to the laboratory. These samples mirror the urine samples that establishments send away for testing. The establishment is advised subsequently by Tackler Analytical which samples have been sent to the laboratory and which barcodes have been used to identify them. A confirmation test is requested by the prison on any sample which screens positive, using the normal procedure and once the confirmation test results are received back in the establishment the results are faxed back to Tackler Analytical.

By adopting the Blind Performance Challenge Programme, the Prison Service can safeguard both the quality and integrity of the mandatory drug testing process.

Quality assurance

No screening system can guarantee 100 per cent results, but the safeguard with MDT is the opportunity to request a confirmation test. That both a screening test and a confirmation test exist allows prisoners subject to disciplinary proceedings an opportunity to challenge the laboratory results. If they remain dissatisfied in the final analysis, prisoners can request that a sample is sent away for independent laboratory analysis.

Understandably no dip and read testing kit or on-site screening machine can match this degree of accuracy or guarantee the results to be consistently accurate. Dip and read testing is the methodology chosen for voluntary drug testing. The results of a voluntary drug test do not in isolation carry the same weight as the results of those samples tested under the mandatory drug testing programme under quality-assured laboratory conditions. Dip and read testing alone does not provide evidence of drug misuse beyond reasonable doubt. This has implications for the way in which prisons implement compacts, and the way they administer the Incentive and Earned Privilege Scheme on voluntary testing units.

TAKING DISCIPLINARY ACTION

Disciplinary hearings are held by the Governor (or Controller in a privately run prison), on a daily basis, except for Sundays and statutory or public holidays. The hearings are investigative, while the court system is adversarial. The Governor's primary role is to determine whether the prisoner is guilty of the offence charged, establish the facts, find out what really happened and the reasons for the breach of discipline. The process must be conducted fairly with proper regard to the principles of natural justice and the Governor must be impartial. Hearings are held as soon as practical and within 48 hours of the charge being discovered. Justice delayed is justice denied. 'Justice in prison [should be] secured through the exercise of responsibility and respect. The achievement of justice will itself enhance security and control,' said Lord Justice Woolf in the Woolf Report 1991.

Laying charges

Once the prisoner has been issued with Form 1127, Notice of Report, he must be given a minimum of two hours to prepare his answer to the charge. Prisoners charged under Prison Rule 51 paragraph 9, YOI Rule 50 paragraph 8A, 'administers a controlled drug to himself or fails to prevent the administration of a controlled drug to him by another person' – must be issued with a sheet entitled Information for Prisoners who have Tested Positive for Drugs. This follows a judgment in the Divisional Court in 1998 when the policy on MDT adjudications was challenged at judicial review.

Prior to the hearing, the medical officer will examine the prisoner and satisfy himself he is mentally fit to plead and, if found guilty of the charge, is physically fit to undergo punishment, particularly if a period of time in cellular confinement is awarded by the Governor.

Following examination, the medical officer signs a certification of medical fitness on Form F256, the Record of Hearing and Adjudication, on which the adjudicating Governor makes a formal record of the hearing and outcome, including the punishment he decides is appropriate.

Although Governors' adjudications are a formal occasion, they should be conducted in a relaxed atmosphere and prisoners must be allowed to sit during the proceedings and be given writing materials in order to make notes. Escorting staff sit either side of the inmate, but are not allowed to face him (known as 'eyeballing') during the proceedings; this practice is intimidatory and inhibits the accused when conducting their defence. If eyeballing does occur, there are grounds for complaint to the Area Manager under the Request and Complaint system, and the adjudication will be quashed under Prison Rule 61 or YOI Rule 59. The procedure at the adjudication is laid out on Form 1145, Explanation of Procedure at Disciplinary Charge Hearings, which is given to the inmate at the same time as Form 1127.

If the prisoner pleads guilty to the offence, the reporting officer reads out the evidence from Form F254, Report to the Governor of Alleged Offence by Inmate. The accused is given the opportunity to question the evidence or comment upon it – he may request a witness to corroborate his version of events. If a written answer to the charge is made, this will be read out during the hearing and the inmate may be asked questions by the Governor.

Mitigating circumstances

Once the Governor is satisfied that the charge has been proved beyond a reasonable doubt, he will invite the prisoner to make a plea of mitigation. This provides an opportunity for any explanation for poor behaviour to be considered, or for relevant family or medical problems to be highlighted.

Prisoners pleading guilty may find it preferable and advantageous to make a statement of mitigation on the back of Form F1127.

Conduct reports

Following the plea of mitigation, a member of staff from the Segregation Unit will read out a conduct report which has been prepared by wing staff. It will explain to the Governor how the accused has behaved and cooperated with staff while in custody. However, the wing report must not comment on any previous convictions or refer to any previous periods of custody served. The prisoner then has the opportunity to comment upon the conduct report

Responding to the charge

If no plea or a not guilty plea is entered, the reporting officer will read out a statement and the prisoner will be given the opportunity to ask questions or comment on the evidence. The Governor will question the officer and any other witnesses that are called. The prisoner will also have the opportunity to question any witnesses.

The prisoner can also request witnesses. Normally, witnesses will be called if they are willing to attend, and they may have relevant evidence. The Governor has a discretion to refuse to call witnesses but this discretion must be exercised reasonably and on proper grounds, for example, if it is clear that the witness has no relevant evidence.

Once all the witnesses have appeared and the accused given the opportunity to question them, he has a further opportunity to say anything additional in his defence.

Once the evidence has been heard, the Governor has to decide whether the charge has been proved beyond reasonable doubt. He will listen to any mitigation the inmate wishes to be considered, then request a conduct report and decide on an appropriate punishment.

Proceeding in the accused's absence

The hearing will proceed in the accused's absence if he fails to cooperate by refusing to attend, being indecently dressed or by being in a condition that is offensive to the adjudicator, for example, on a dirty protest. He will be advised that the hearing will go ahead in spite of his failure to cooperate. If this happens, a not guilty plea will be entered and the fact that the accused did not attend the hearing will be noted on Form F256, the Record of Hearing and Adjudication. Following a recent judicial review where an inmate claimed he had been refused permission to attend an adjudication, the following information is recorded on the F256:

1. that the accused has been seen and informed that the hearing will proceed in his absence;
2. the name of the person who spoke to the accused;
3. what the accused said in response.

The prisoner will be advised of the outcome of the hearing, invited to offer any mitigation, then informed of the punishment.

CONDUCTING A DEFENCE

Any prisoner who feels unable to conduct his defence without assistance can request, when he attends the hearing, legal representation, or an adviser or friend, to be present.

Although prisoners can request legal representation, there is no right of representation and such requests are, in fact, rarely granted. The level of disciplinary awards has been reduced since the Board of Visitors (BoV) was removed from the internal disciplinary process. At one time, the BoV could impose a punishment of 180 additional days, equivalent to a further twelve months' sentence before remission is taken into account. Governors' powers, whilst more limited, are significant – an additional 42 days is equivalent to a three-month sentence in the local magistrate's court.

Requesting legal representation

In considering any request for legal representation, the adjudicator must consider the following criteria:

- the seriousness of the charge and the potential penalty;
- if any points of law are likely to arise;
- the ability of the prisoner to present his case;
- whether there are likely to be procedural difficulties;
- the need for reasonable speed in completing his adjudication;
- the need for fairness between prisoners and prison staff, particularly when there are several co-accused.

A prisoner can also request access to legal advice (as distinct from legal representation). Such access must be granted unless there are good grounds for refusing it.

A further option is for an inmate to request the assistance of an adviser or friend, often referred to as a McKenzie man. His role is to take notes and offer advice, but he is not entitled to take part in the proceedings or speak on behalf of the accused unless invited to by the Governor.

LEGAL DEFENCES

An adjudicator must be *satisfied beyond reasonable doubt* that an offence against discipline has been committed. An important element that needs to be established is *intent* on the part of the accused. For example, in the case of a charge of being in possession of any unauthorized article (Rule 51, paragraph 12), there are three elements that need to be fully satisfied. First, presence – that the article exists and can be produced; second, knowledge – that the inmate knew it was where it was discovered and third, control – that the offending article was owned by the accused and was under his personal control.

The Prison Rules 1999 set out, in Rule 52, three specific defences to a charge laid under Rule 51(9): 'administers a controlled drug to himself or fails to prevent the administration of a controlled drug to him by another person'. Legitimate defences to this charge are for the inmate to show that:

(a) the controlled drug had been prior to its administration lawfully in his possession for his use or was administered to him in the course of a lawful supply of the drug to him by another person;
(b) the controlled drug was administered by or to him in circumstances in which he did not know and had no reason to suspect that such a drug was being administered;
(c) the controlled drug was administered by or to him under duress or to him without consent in circumstances where it was not reasonable for him to have resisted.

The wording of the charge Rule 51(9), and the existence of these specific defences to the charge, clarifies the burden of proof necessary to reach a guilty verdict. In the absence of a credible explanation from the inmate or a witness, the adjudicator can arrive at a finding of guilt based on the positive test result, and does not need to have any other additional evidence as to knowledge or intent.

A further defence that can be offered is if the accused has been charged with using the same drug within the minimum waiting periods (see p. 68). Once an alleged offence has been committed under this rule, two elements have to be established. First, that an initial screening test has given a positive result and second, that at all material times, the inmate was in prison custody when the drug was administered. If the controlled drug was taken whilst on temporary release (in accordance with Rule 9), then the inmate would be charged with failing to comply with the conditions of temporary licence, which prohibits the use of a controlled drug.

Challenging the confirmation test

Although the confirmation test report is clearly hearsay evidence, it is an exception to the normal restrictions on the use of hearsay evidence because in the criminal courts there is provision to treat expert evidence differently. This contention was challenged in the Divisional Court in May 1998, when a prisoner called Wynter argued at judicial review that the laboratory scientist must be called as a witness if a prisoner wishes to challenge the findings contained in the confirmation test report. The Divisional Court confirmed that the laboratory reports are hearsay evidence, but agreed that the confirmation test report could continue to be admitted as evidence, even when a prisoner disputes the test results and the laboratory scientist is not called as a witness. The court did state that establishments should provide prisoners with more information about the test and the testing process, which would lessen demands for the attendance of the laboratory scientist. This is contained in a five-page information sheet titled 'Information for Prisoners Who Have Tested Positive for Drugs', issued to all inmates charged under Rule 51(9).

Requesting a professional witness

Prisoners who make a request for the laboratory scientist have to satisfy the adjudicating Governor as to why they wish the witness to be called and what relevant evidence the witness can give in addition to that contained in the confirmation test report.

A refusal to call the witness must be made on proper grounds which should be recorded on the F256 Record of Hearing and Adjudication. Inconvenience and expense are not legitimate reasons for failing to call a witness and are grounds for appeal.

Should the adjudicator decide to call the relevant laboratory scientist, because he considers there is a legitimate challenge to the scientific evidence, for example a conflicting report from independent analysis, the case should be adjourned to be discussed and investigated. The Drug Strategy Unit in Headquarters should make the necessary arrangements with the laboratory concerned.

GOVERNORS' PUNISHMENTS

If the Governor finds a prisoner guilty of an offence he can impose one or more of the following punishments under Rule 55 of The Prison Rules 1999 in the case of adults and under Rule 57 in the case of Young Offenders under the age of 21 when the offence was committed:

(a) caution;

(b) loss of privileges for a maximum period of 42 days (21 days if under 21);

(c) exclusion from associated work for up to 21 days (adults only);

(d) stoppage of or deduction from earnings for up to 84 days and of an amount of up to 42 days' earnings (the maximum period of stoppage of or deduction from earnings shall be 42 days and the maximum amount shall be 21 days if under 21);

(e) cellular confinement for up to 14 days (7 days if under 21). Adjudicators may not give a punishment of cellular confinement to any prisoner who was under 18 years of age at the time the offence was committed.

(f) up to a maximum of 42 added days to the sentence. However, additional days are not available as a punishment for any prisoner who is serving a period of detention under a Detention and Training Order.

(g) forfeit for any period of the right to have their own books, newspapers, writing materials and other means of occupation (in the case of an unconvicted prisoner only).

Any punishment can be suspended for up to six months (Rule 60) and a prospective award of additional days can be given to a prisoner who is detained on remand and which takes effect only if the inmate in question is subsequently sentenced (Rule 59).

No one must undergo a punishment of cellular confinement until the medical officer has certified that there are no medical reasons why the prisoner should not do so (Rule 58). Anyone serving a punishment of cellular confinement must be kept in a cell that contains as a minimum a bed, bedding, a table and stool or chair.

If the inmate is found guilty of more than one charge arising from an incident, the punishment can be ordered to run consecutively. In the case of additional days the overall maximum must not exceed 42 days and cellular confinement must not exceed 14 days (Rule 55).

Governors are obliged to provide local guidelines to adjudicators for each offence which set out the range of penalties for particular offences within their establishments, in order to ensure consistency between different adjudicating Governors.

A new clause (Prison Rule 55(4) and YOI Rule 53(4) added to The Prison Rules 1999) requires the Governor to 'take into account any guidelines that the Secretary of State may from time to time issue as to the level of punishment that should normally be imposed for a particular offence'. In the case of offences involving receiving drugs through visits or an unauthorized transaction in visits, the Secretary of State has approved guidelines which Governors are obliged to follow.

ADJUDICATION GUIDELINES

In April 1999, new procedures were introduced to cover incidents of drug smuggling or prisoners receiving drugs on a visit. They included the level of adjudication awards. Prison Rule 55(4) and YOI Rule 53(4) require Governors to take into account guidelines approved by the Secretary of State when deciding on a punishment: 'In imposing a punishment, the Governor shall take into account any guidelines that the Secretary of State may from time to time issue as to the level of punishment that should normally be imposed for a particular offence against discipline'. These guidelines are based on the level of punishments that Governors awarded throughout 1997 for the offence of possessing an unauthorized drug.

Punishment levels

Adult males, adult females, young offenders (both male and female), juvenile and unconvicted or unsentenced prisoners are to be treated within the parameters shown in the following table.

Table 1: Punishment levels

Award	Level	Notes
(a) ADDITIONAL DAYS	8–14 days	Either alone or combined with other punishments
(b) FORFEITURE OF PRIVILEGES	1–7 days	Combined with other punishments
(c) STOPPAGE OF EARNINGS	1–7 days	Combined with other punishments
(d) CELLULAR CONFINEMENT	1–7 days	Combined with additional days. Not available as a punishment for any prisoner who was under 18 years of age at the time the offence was committed
Lifers only		
(e) STOPPAGE OF EARNINGS	8–14 days	Combined with other punishments
(f) FORFEITURE OF PRIVILEGES	1–7 days	Combined with other punishments
(g) CELLULAR CONFINEMENT	7 days	Either alone or combined with stoppage of earnings

Note: Any award of additional days to unconvicted/unsentenced prisoners must be prospective added days. Additional days are not available as a punishment for any prisoner who is serving a period of detention under a Detention and Training Order.

Mitigating and aggravating factors

Adjudicators still have considerable discretion to use their judgement, and can vary the awards and depart from the ranges quoted in the guidelines where the circumstances warrant it.

Mitigating factors
- first offence;
- class C drug;

- small quantity of an unauthorized class C drug (personal use);
- where the prisoner is actively seeking help to address his drug addiction by being on a voluntary testing unit or involved in voluntary testing, or attending a Drug Awareness/Substance Group;
- under pressure to smuggle drugs for another prisoner;
- physical and mental health factors;
- expresses remorse, is open and cooperative;
- age and level of maturity (particularly with youngsters).

Aggravating factors
- pattern of similar offences;
- dealing in class B or C drugs;
- possession of a class A drug;
- dealing in class A drugs.

Mandatory frequent testing

Since August 1999, any prisoners found guilty at an adjudication of misusing a class A drug, such as opiates, cocaine, methadone or LSD, are automatically placed on a programme of mandatory frequent urine testing. This means that each month they will be targeted for an MDT test (the number of frequent tests to be decided by the Governors) and a further positive result will mean another disciplinary charge.

CASE STUDY

John is selected for a random test

John is selected by computer for random testing and is taken to the drug-testing centre where he is asked to provide a sample. He is handed a Mandatory Drug Test Authorization Form which advises him he has been selected for the test on a strictly random basis. It explains the procedure being followed and points out the consequences of failing to provide a sample within four hours or, exceptionally, five hours. He is invited to sign the Consent to Medical Disclosure and declare that he has not used any medication issued to him by health care. He produces a sample of urine in the receptacle provided and is then handed the Prison Service Chain of Custody Procedure Form, which sets out the seventeen stages in the procedure which have to be followed and is asked to confirm the sample was processed according to laid-down procedure.

Once the sample has been provided, it is divided into two tubes, sealed with tamper proof seals and placed into the chain of custody bag. John is advised to return to his wing and told he will be called up and advised of the results as soon as the sample returns to the establishment from the laboratory.

The urine sample is given an initial screening test at the laboratory and the result turns out to be negative. John is advised of the outcome and given a certificate which confirms he tested negative.

CHECKLIST

- Has a serious criminal offence been committed that warrants referral to the police and is in the public interest for a prosecution to proceed? The following offences meet this criteria:
  (a) possession with or without intent to supply a Class A drug;
  (b) possession with intent to supply a Class B drug.
- Was the charge laid within 48 hours of discovering the alleged offence?
- Does the test result indicate a controlled drug is present in the urine sample?
- Were the mandatory drug testing procedures followed correctly?
- Has a significant irregularity occurred in the chain of custody? The following would invalidate the integrity of the process:
  (a) only one bottle placed in the sample bag;
  (b) an insufficient quantity of urine sample;
  (c) a broken/tampered seal on a sample bottle or on the chain of custody bag;
  (d) any leakage from a sample bottle in transit;
  (e) an inconsistency in the barcodes between the sample bottles and the chain of custody form;
  (f) a failure by the officer taking the sample to sign the declaration stating the correct procedure has been followed.
- Was the prisoner in custody under Prison Rules or YOI Rules when the drug was allegedly taken?
- Were the minimum waiting periods, after first reception and between samples for the same drug, observed?
- Does prima facie evidence exist that the drug was administered under duress or taken without the inmate's knowledge?
- Was the controlled drug lawfully prescribed by the medical officer?
- Has appropriate action been taken in response to a positive screening test in respect of the following drugs?
  (a) *Cannabis*
     Medical information is completely unnecessary, and a confirmation test is only required if the prisoner pleads not guilty.
  (b) *Cocaine and LSD*
     Medical information is required if the prisoner pleads not guilty, and a confirmation test is only required if the prisoner pleads not guilty.

(c) *Methadone, benzodiazepines and barbiturates*

These are controlled drugs that can be prescribed legally. Medical information is required immediately after screening positive. A confirmation test is highly unlikely to distinguish between prescribed drugs and drug misuse.

(d) *Opiates and amphetamines*

Some drugs that are codeine-based painkillers or cough mixtures can give a positive screening result for opiates or amphetamines, therefore medical information is required at an early stage following receipt of a positive test result. The outcome of a confirmation test can be obtained before a charge is laid.

(e) *All drugs*

The onus is on the prisoner to provide credible evidence that a positive test result is due to prescribed medicine. A refusal to give permission for medical disclosure can result in a legitimate finding of guilt.

- Has the charge been proved *beyond reasonable doubt,* meaning that no credible evidence, sufficiently strong to raise more than a doubt in the adjudicator's mind, has been produced?
- Was the prisoner given an opportunity to explain his or her actions and say anything in mitigation?

CHAPTER 6

Reducing Demand for Drugs

THE TREATMENT OF DRUG MISUSERS

The CARAT process for remand and sentenced prisoners is now in place. The CARAT service provider can be a specialist drug worker, trained prison officer, health care specialist or probation officer. He raises a casework record on every prisoner who comes into contact with CARAT services. This initial contact can be on reception or at the induction stage. However, a referral for services can be made at any stage during the sentence, or any time whilst held on remand.

The objective is to provide a complete picture of all the work that is undertaken to address a prisoner's drug problem. This ensures that continuity of care is maintained when a prisoner is transferred to another prison or YOI. At that point, the CARAT team in that establishment can provide ongoing support and work in line with the agreed care plan.

Referral for CARAT services

Any prisoner identified with a drug problem can be referred to the CARAT team by prison staff, who complete a simple referral form. Contact is then quickly made with the prisoner and advice and information made available to them regarding their drug use.

Following this initial contact it can be determined whether the prisoner has a problem with drugs and if it is appropriate to carry out a full assessment.

COORDINATING THE APPROACH

A full CARAT assessment should be carried out within five working days of initial contact. This involves obtaining a range of reports from other agencies in order to make a comprehensive assessment of the prisoner's needs. Although it is essential to gain a complete picture of the prisoner's involvement with outside agencies, the CARAT worker must obtain the consent of the prisoner to the transfer of confidential information.

Sharing confidential information

Prisoners are asked to sign a Prisoner's Consent to the Transfer of Information form which allows a CARAT worker to obtain confidential information about their medical and social background from other agencies.

The consent form includes a declaration expressed in the terms shown in Figure 5.

Principles of confidentiality

The following principles apply to the sharing of confidential information:

- respect for the prisoner's wishes;
- information is shared after discussion about what is necessary and who needs access to this information;
- the safety and security of other prisoners and staff is paramount and cannot be compromised by not revealing information;
- if the prisoner is transferred, he is advised that the casework record is being passed on to the CARAT team at the new establishment;
- prisoner confidentiality is respected subject to security, child care and self-harm restraints;
- the CARAT worker is committed to promoting the concept of collaborative work and sharing information on the basis of making informed decisions;
- the issue of disclosure extends to third parties which means that the CARAT worker obtains the written consent of the third party before disclosing information to the prisoner or other staff.

These principles are all subject to the interests of the security of the establishment being paramount, the requirements of existing child care legislation, and the prevention of self-harm or suicide.

Making a full assessment

The CARAT worker completing the CARAT assessment form tries to obtain as many reports as possible that can help him to understand the prisoner's drug problem. Naturally he need not duplicate requests for reports that are requested by the establishment in the normal course of events by other departments. For instance, the Observation Classification and Allocation (OCA) unit has a responsibility to obtain external reports about previous convictions, details of charges, pleas, findings and sentence details relating to the current offence.

Should the current concerns about the prisoner be primarily about their psychological health and potential suicidal behaviour, an immediate referral to health care using the F2052SH Self-Harm at Risk form may be necessary.

Once interviews have been conducted, relevant reports consulted and a comprehensive assessment completed, the CARAT worker should discuss with the prisoner his assessment of the main factors he believes contribute to the prisoner's drug problem, the drug treatment options available to the prisoner, and the likely outcomes the prisoner expects will result from the proposed course of action.

The following information is intended to make you aware of what can happen to the things said between yourself and your CARAT team and therefore to help you to decide what you do and do not want to be known. Sharing the right information with the right people who have and who may be involved in helping you can be beneficial.

There can be good reasons however why you may not want some people or groups of people to know what you have been discussing. Under these circumstances you will also need to know whether this will prevent the drug worker from helping you in any way. At the outset of any contact with a CARAT worker, s/he will explain this to you and help you to decide how much about yourself you want to tell others.

Before information is requested from or passed on to another agency or discipline, your CARAT team will talk with you about the information which needs to be passed on in connection with your treatment. You will be asked to sign the following agreement to the exchange of information with other professionals involved with your care.

If you decide you do not wish the CARAT team to share information about you this will be respected **unless**:

*   the safety and security of the prison and those within it, both prisoners and staff is compromised by not revealing information;

*   your CARAT team believes you may be at risk of self-harm; or

*   your CARAT team has concerns under the Children Act 1989 eg. the welfare of any children who may be in your care.

A CARAT worker has discussed with me the purposes and benefits of sharing information about issues related to my drug use and the work undertaken to address these issues with other people, issues which remain confidential, and the limits to confidentiality.

I understand that communication between staff and outside agencies is intended to support me in making changes.

I give permission for my CARAT worker, ..., to receive any information about me from or to provide any information to:

(a)	My GP in the community	(i)	My Personal Officer
(b)	My Doctor/nurse/counsellor at the DDU	(j)	Bail Information Officer
(c)	Community agency drug counsellor	(k)	Pre-Sentence Report Writer
(d)	My home Probation Officer	(l)	Chaplaincy
(e)	Community Care Assessor	(m)	My family
(f)	Prison Doctor/nurse/healthcare staff	(n)	My solicitor
(g)	Probation Staff in prison	(o)	Other CARAT workers
(h)	Prison Officers (eg. Sentence Planning)	(p)	Other (specify)

If you do not wish your CARAT worker to speak to any of the above people, you should cross through that person and add your initials.

Prisoner's signature   Date

CARAT worker to note names, addresses and contact numbers on Contacts Sheet.

Figure 5: Prisoner's Consent to the Transfer of Information form

Once the prisoner has seen the completed assessment, he is invited to sign the document. The next stage in the process is to prepare and agree a care plan with the prisoner, within ten days of completing the full assessment.

ASSESSING TREATMENT NEEDS

Once a full assessment has been completed, the CARAT worker should have a clear picture of the problem areas facing the prisoner, and he should know of what available courses of treatment can address the identified needs.

The care plan sets out clear goals and objectives to achieve and identifies what needs to be done, by whom and when. It evaluates whether the goals have been achieved in the agreed timescale.

The CARAT worker considers all the treatment options including one-to-one counselling, groupwork, attending a rehabilitation programme or referral to a VTU with ongoing CARAT support.

Setting effective targets

All targets agreed between the prisoner and the CARAT worker much be SMART, that is:

- **S**pecific
  The targets must not be vague or aspirational, but expressed in clear, unambiguous, succinct terms.
- **M**easurable
  Only drug-related targets are set where progress is capable of being achieved within an agreed timetable. Specific objectives are agreed, such as attending a drug awareness course or gaining admission to a voluntary testing unit.
- **A**chievable
  Targets must be achieved during the current sentence or after release whilst under supervision on licence.
- **R**ealistic
  It is important that all parties appreciate that every identified need cannot be met. Some targets are only capable of fulfilment in the long term, whereas others are achievable in the short term. Some depend on the availability of resources, such as a rehabilitation programme which may only be available in another establishment.
- **T**ime-bounded
  A realistic timescale for achieving each target is agreed where progress is monitored on a regular basis by the prisoner and CARAT worker.

A multi-disciplinary framework

The importance of regular liaison with other service providers in the prison or YOI cannot be over-emphasized. Issues such as employment needs, accommodation, education, training requirements and potential resettlement problems need to be anticipated, so that a coordinated action plan can be devised.

Close cooperation between the CARAT worker and those involved in the sentence management process is necessary, with the CARAT worker providing a report for the initial sentence plan and any sentence plan reviews held.

The prisoner agrees and signs the care plan and is given a copy. The care plan is copied and sent to the external probation officer and any outside agencies involved. If a prisoner is involved in sentence management, their personal officer also receives a copy, providing the prisoner gives his consent to the transfer of information.

Preparing a release plan

The release plan summarizes the main issues tackled in custody and identifies the prisoner's main achievements prior to release. It covers the prisoner's drug use prior to CARAT's involvement and charts the progress made in custody. The main priorities for work after release are identified, as are the arrangements for continuing treatment, and which community drug agency is involved in the throughcare.

The release plan prepared for prisoners on remand is part of an overall package produced for the courts. It includes details of all the options available in the community, so that alternatives to custody can be considered.

The CARAT team liaise with, and provide a report to, the prison probation officer whose role is to prepare a risk assessment for the Home Detention Board on all prisoners eligible for Home Detention Curfew.

The CARAT release plan contributes to the overall sentence management release plan and has a bearing on decisions relating to Release on Temporary Licence (ROTL), Discretionary Conditional Release (DCR) and parole. In the case of prisoners serving a life sentence, it can impact on the licence conditions that are being considered to reduce further any risk to the public.

Ongoing work in custody is discontinued if there is agreement between the CARAT worker and the prisoner that there is no longer a need to address drug issues.

Post-release

An important responsibility of the CARAT worker is to help prisoners gain access to community services. This is a major obstacle since there are often waiting lists to negotiate and resistance to overcome about giving any priority to ex-prisoners.

After release the CARAT worker may continue offering aftercare for a maximum of eight weeks, where access to a community-based agency cannot be obtained. If the discharge address is at a distance, arrangements are made to provide support with a community-based agency. Once the discharge prisoner has attended an appointment with the external agency, further involvement by the CARAT team ceases.

REMAND PRISONERS

Figure 6 should be examined in conjunction with these explanatory notes.

1. *Prisoner received in prison.*
2. *Given health care assessment on reception.*
   If a drug problem is identified he is referred for CARAT services or for detoxification.

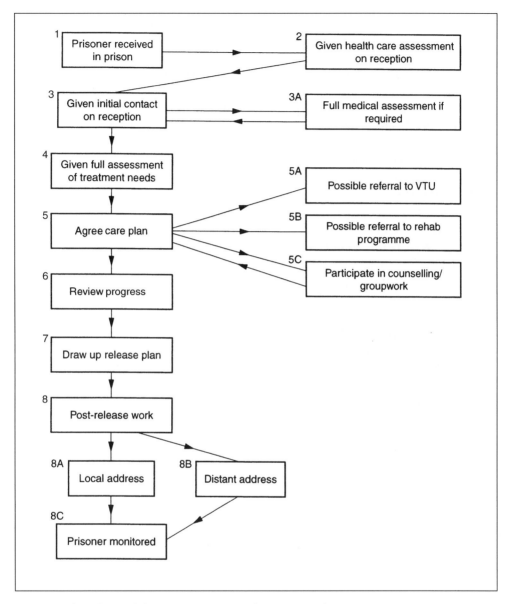

Figure 6: Flowchart of the CARAT process for a remand prisoner

3. *Given initial contact on reception.*
   On reception, advice and information is provided by a CARAT worker.
3A. *Full medical assessment if required.*
   Relevant information is obtained from community health agencies.
4. *Given full assessment of treatment needs.*
   Consent is obtained to contact other agencies, including external drug agencies and the Probation Service.

A full assessment of the prisoner's needs is made within five working days of the initial referral.

On request, this assessment is provided to defence solicitors, the Crown Prosecution Service, bail information officers and community drug agencies.

5.   *Agree care plan.*
The agreed care plan is produced within ten working days of the full assessment and copied to Probation and other community agencies involved.

5A. *Possible referral to VTU.*

5B. *Possible referral to rehabilitation programme.*

5C. *Participate in counselling/groupwork.*

6.   *Review progress.*
Progress and goals are reviewed and new review dates set.

7.   *Draw up release plan.*
The CARAT release plan is developed as part of a package for the court and the Probation Service are advised if a community sentence is being proposed.

The prisoner is helped to access community services on release.

8.   *Post-release work.*

8A. *Local address.*
Where prisoners are released to a local address, supervision continues for up to eight weeks after discharge.

If they are not under probation supervision at this point, they are transferred to a community-based agency.

8B. *Distant address.*
Where the prisoner is released to a distant address, liaison takes place to ensure initial contact is made between the prisoner and a community-based drug agency.

8C. *Prisoner monitored.*
Post-release monitoring takes place up until initial contact is made with an external agency.

SENTENCED PRISONERS

Figure 7 should be examined in conjunction with these explanatory notes.

1.   *Prisoner received in prison.*

2.   *Given health care assessment on reception.*
If a drug problem is identified, he is referred for CARAT services or for detoxification.

3.   *Given initial contact on reception or induction.*
On reception, advice and information is given by a CARAT worker.

3A. *Possible full medical assessment.*
Relevant information is obtained from community health agencies.

4.   *Given full assessment of treatment needs.*
Consent is obtained to contact other agencies, including external drug agencies and the Probation Service.

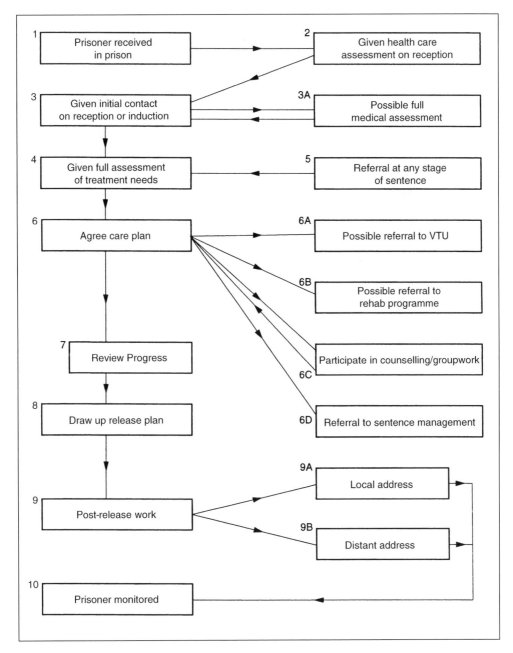

Figure 7: Flowchart of the CARAT process for a sentenced prisoner

A full assessment of the prisoner's needs is made within five working days of initial contact or detoxification.

5. *Referral at any stage of sentence.*
   This can be self-referral, a result of a pre-sentence report, following a positive MDT, or a result of the sentence management process.

6.   *Agree care plan.*
     The agreed care plan is produced within ten working days of the full assessment
     and, as part of the sentence management process, is copied to the personal officer.
6A. *Possible referral to VTU.*
6B. *Possible referral to rehabilitation programme.*
6C. *Participate in counselling/groupwork.*
6D. *Referral to sentence management.*
     Prisoners serving longer sentences are referred to sentence management following
     completion of CARAT.
7.   *Review progress.*
     Progress and goals are reviewed and the care plan fed into sentence management
     process.
8.   *Draw up release plan.*
     The CARAT release plan contributes to the overall sentence management release
     plan and the prisoner is helped to gain access to services in the community on
     discharge.
          The Probation Service is notified of prisoners released on licence.
          The release plan of prisoners eligible for Home Detention Curfew is sent to the
     prison probation officer and relevant community drug agency.
9.   *Post-release work.*
9A. *Local address.*
     Where a prisoner is released to a local address, supervision can continue for up to
     eight weeks after discharge, if a community-based agency has not assumed
     responsibility.
          If they are not under probation supervision at this point, they are transferred
     to a community-based agency.
9B. *Distant address.*
     Where the prisoner is released to a distant address, liaison takes place to ensure
     initial contact is made between the prisoner and a community-based drug agency;
     if not possible, there is nothing to stop telephone contact being maintained.
9C. *Prisoner monitored.*
     Post-release monitoring takes place to ensure the first appointment with the
     external agency is kept.

VOLUNTARY TESTING UNITS (VTUs)

The policy document 'Tackling Drugs in Prison' has as its third aim: 'to enable people
with drug problems to overcome them and live healthy and crime free lives'. The
Prison Service is committed to giving all prisoners access to voluntary testing and
establishing voluntary testing units alongside a range of treatment opportunities
suitable for offenders.

The Annual Report for the Prison Service (1998–9) clearly states:

Increased emphasis is being placed on providing support for prisoners who
make a commitment to remain drug free by setting up voluntary testing units.

It is intended by the year 2001 to have sufficient voluntary testing spaces for all suitable prisoners who request a place. Part of the CSR funding will be allocated to develop this necessary infrastructure in support of this initiative.

The Woolf Report

The idea of voluntary testing units is by no means new. The Woolf Report (January 1991), which enquired into the riots that took place in 1990, reported that drug abuse was widespread. This claim was supported by research that demonstrated the following figures on substance abuse:

* 20.1% of the adult male sentenced population;
* 15.8% of sentenced male young prisoners;
* 28.9% of sentenced female prisoners.

Woolf cited good practice in other countries and concluded that the Prison Service should take every opportunity to make treatment available to prisoners: 'In the Netherlands, there are drug-free units in some prisons where an improved regime is offered to prisoners who agree to participate in programmes. Similar units could be created here.' He made several recommendations in his forward-looking report, some of which are now happening:

* *Staff training*
  Training of prison staff should be improved.
* *Detoxification*
  A standard opiate withdrawal regime should be introduced.
* *Therapeutic communities*
  Therapeutic community treatment should be provided.
* *Throughcare*
  There should be close liaison with community groups as part of a prisoner's release plan.

The Learmont Report

This made two specific recommendations about tackling drug abuse:

1. The concept of drug-free wings and of drug testing should be implemented where appropriate (Recommendation 84).
2. To deal with drug abuse, all prisons must have programmes that inform, educate and help prisoners combat the drug habit. Success on such programmes should be rewarded through the incentive scheme (Recommendation 85).

Drug-free wings and mandatory drug testing offers some protection, particularly to those afraid of becoming a victim of the drug culture, and may help to isolate those who gain power from drug trafficking.

Drug Misuse in Prison

The strategy document 'Drug Misuse in Prison' was positive about the potential value of voluntary testing units, which it envisaged as an interim step towards the longer-term goal of eradicating drugs in prison.

The concept of VTUs is based on European practice where special areas or wings are set up for prisoners who agree not to use drugs and are willing to undergo regular random urine testing. The idea is to support and actively encourage prisoners who agree to stay off drugs during their sentence and address their drug misuse or drug-dependency problem.

Those who complete drug treatment programmes sign compacts not to take drugs whilst living in a voluntary testing unit. Should they fail to abide by the terms of the compact, sanctions can be applied against them under the Incentive and Earned Privilege System.

THE VERNE EXPERIENCE

In June 1996, HMP The Verne set up a voluntary testing unit. In 1998, it held a workshop to share its experiences. There had been several problems setting up the VTU because tactical management considerations meant that the wing had to be kept full at all times and additional funding to set up the unit was not available. Despite these difficulties compacts were introduced and a system of incentives and earned privileges developed, which included a range of activities, including quizzes, bingo, pool, table tennis and karaoke.

Aims of the VTU

The published aims of the VTU at HMP The Verne are:

* to provide a safe, substance-free environment;
* to provide training, support and encouragement for prisoners wishing to overcome substance misuse problems;
* to reduce health risks associated with substance misuse;
* to reduce the risks of further offending as a result of substance misuse.

The following criteria were developed in order to decide which prisoners to admit onto the unit:

* those with a drug/alcohol problem who are actively seeking help;
* those wishing to be drug/alcohol free and who are willing to agree to a policy of complete abstinence;
* those willing to undertake voluntary drug testing.

Drug testing

A drug-testing machine was obtained from Behring Diagnostics UK Ltd which uses the Enzyme Multiplied Immunoassay Technique (EMIT). This involves the use of antibodies and enzymes to produce Nictinamide Adenine Dinucleotide (NAD) which is checked for absorbency of light.

The machine makes checks and gives each sample a numerical value which is compared to the benchmark set into the machine. If the number is equal to or higher than the benchmark, then the sample is positive. Conversely, if the number is lower than the benchmark, the sample is negative.

It is important that the machine is carefully calibrated and maintained by a qualified operator. Calibration is carried out using known amounts of the substances that are tested to get an accurate level.

The Verne discovered that having a drug-testing machine on the VTU dramatically improved the effectiveness of the unit. In 1996, 178 tests were carried out, of which 107 were negative and 71 positive. This is 39.8 per cent testing positive with some testing positive for more than one drug. Of the 71 who tested positive, 46 were positive for cannabis, 25 for opiates and 8 for benzodiazepines.

In 1997, 678 tests were carried out, of which 453 were negative and 225 were positive. This is 33.1 per cent testing positive with some testing positive for more than one drug. Of the 225 who tested positive, 146 were positive for cannabis, 77 were positive for opiates and 26 for benzodiazepines.

Delivering treatment programmes

Counselling services were provided by the Alchemy Project but are currently provided by Cranstoun Drug Services. The treatment programme consisted of twenty half-day groups which were based on the first five steps of the Minnesota twelve-step programme (see p. 121 and Glossary for more details). Since May 1998, the counselling services have developed a multi-disciplinary approach by significantly increasing the number of counsellors and involving prison officers in the delivery of groups.

A structured training programme was put in place that includes presentational skills, group working, basic counselling skills, motivational interviewing techniques and health and safety training. It was supplemented by visits to outside agencies. In addition, some prison officers on the VTU have completed a course accredited by the Open College on Advanced Drug Awareness.

The drug treatment programme for prisoners included:

- a needs assessment;
- educational classes on substance misuse, HIV/AIDS and other health-related issues;
- a treatment programme for prisoners wishing to remain drug-free;
- developing release plans for those with substance misuse problems;
- a referral service to other community-based drug agencies.

There were positive achievements: some prisoners serving long sentences became better equipped to return to society having acquired a range of life skills that enabled them to survive without being drug-dependent. Others continued with drug treatment programmes on release and have maintained a drug-free life style.

The positive benefits

The VTU encouraged better team-working amongst prison staff at The Verne and has improved relationships between staff and prisoners. Discipline on the wing improved and respect for staff has increased. The VTU proved beneficial to prisoners wishing to tackle their drug problems. Demand for places was received from prisoners in other establishments. In April 1999 (the latest available figures), a survey showed that 64 prisons had a VTU or discreet area to conduct testing, with 7,000 places in total available across the prison estate.

These establishments are addressing their drug misuse problems with positive results. The Prison Service is building on these initiatives by propagating best practice and developing its drugs strategy. An example of this is CARATs, which builds on many of these ideas and introduces a consistent approach to addressing drug misuse in all establishments.

VOLUNTARY DRUG TESTING

During 1999, a working group set up by the drug strategy unit in Prison Service headquarters considered how best to meet the operational requirements of the service, achieve value for money and avoid disrupting current voluntary testing methodologies. Their findings were reported in August 1999, after the group had evaluated all the available options for voluntary drug testing, and found urine testing to be the preferred method as it is the most suitable for mass screening. The working group concluded that: 'dip and read testing methodology should be adopted as the method of choice for voluntary testing and that existing SYVA/EMIT systems should be phased out on completion of current contractual arrangements'.

SYVA/EMIT machines used for drugs testing are spread throughout the Prison Service. A widely used model is the SYVA ETS supplied by Behring.

Dip and read testing

The working group feels that dip and read testing has a number of advantages over the available alternatives. These advantages are:

- the system is very flexible and can cope without difficulty with unforeseen increases in demand;
- urine testing costs can be more easily controlled;
- it is more cost-effective in terms of staff training and manpower;
- the adoption of an universal system allows an opportunity to economize by bulk-buying, using central purchasing arrangements;

• many existing SYVA/EMIT machines are not being used efficiently and some are not being used at all.

Dip and read testing should be available on a single-strip basis to reduce costs and allow greater flexibility, but the option to use multi-strip drug testing should be at the discretion of the Governor. (See below for further details on the types of tests.) The working group recommends that a dilution test should be available, but used only on suspicion or at the discretion of the Governor. It advises against adopting a comprehensive internal quality assurance system, since it considers this to be unnecessary given the ethos of voluntary testing units.

Following these deliberations, the drug strategy unit invited tenders to supply dip and read testing kits for the whole service and placed a national contract with EUROMED in April 2000.

The limitations

Dip and read testing and on-site screening machines are suitable for voluntary drug testing in all establishments, but they must not be used for mandatory drug testing. Since such use is unsafe any disciplinary award is open to challenge because the laid-down procedures contained in the *Prison Discipline Manual* have not been followed.

CONDUCTING DIP AND READ TESTS

Dip and read testing is a urine-based immunoassay screening test which can detect amphetamines, cannabis (tetrahydrocannabinol), cocaine and opiates. According to the Substance Abuse and Mental Health Services Administration (SAMHSA), these are the most commonly abused illicit drugs. The most widely abused drugs available on prescription are benzodiazepines, methadone and opiates (morphine).

Types of tests

Tests can be conducted singly using strips or cassettes or as multiple tests using a six drug multiple screening test.

The tester using *strips* first ensures that the urine sample and test device are at room temperature. The testing device is then removed from the foil pouch and dipped into the urine sample for about 30 seconds. This allows the urine sample to travel up the strip. The strip is removed from the sample and the result can be read after ten minutes.

A *cassette* can be used in a similar fashion. When the urine sample and test device are at room temperature, the device is removed from the foil pouch and placed on a clean level surface. Using a pipette, four drops of urine are slowly dispensed into the sample hole of the test device allowing five seconds between each drop. The results can be read after ten minutes.

When conducting *multiple screening tests*, the testing device is inserted into the urine sample for at least one minute. The end of the testing device is placed into the sample of urine up to a depth of 1 cm. The test results can be read after ten minutes.

The results window in the test device clearly displays how two types of enzyme react with a magenta-coloured dye conjugate. The testing device has a control line and a dark reddish-purple line appears if the test is performed correctly.

The test enzymes in the testing device can bind with either a drug metabolite or a dye. When there is no drug present in the sample, the dye in the testing device binds and produces a line. However, if the sample is positive, the drug metabolite blocks the binding sites and prevents a line from forming.

Although a negative result can be read in as little as one or two minutes, the full development time of ten minutes is necessary for a positive result.

Limitations of dip and read tests

Dip and read testing is purely a screening test to indicate the presence of an illegal substance. It cannot provide the tester with a measurement of concentration levels in the urine sample.

These testing devices are claimed by the manufacturers to be highly accurate. A confirmation test service is available in the manufacturers' laboratories if required.

False readings can occur if there are contaminates in the sample, such as bleach and strong oxidizing agents.

Certain cough medicines, products used to counter diarrhoea, any medication which contains opiate derivatives, and food compounds which contain poppy seeds taken in large quantities can all produce a positive result.

PRISONER COMPACTS

The idea of having prisoner compacts was originally recommended in the Woolf Report. The Prison Service are committed to their use in all prisons and YOIs.

It is essential to have compacts in place in a voluntary testing unit where prisoner agreement to having voluntary urine tests is an integral part of the regime. This is normally a pre-condition for acceptance onto a VTU.

A prisoner compact is a voluntary agreement freely entered into by both the prisoner and the establishment. It sets out clearly what is expected from prisoners and in return makes plain the facilities and range of privileges available to them. It acts as a powerful incentive to prisoners who wish to conform and earn the right to have an enhanced level of privileges. The compact also sets down what happens if either party fails to keep their side of the agreement.

Although compacts are separate from the prisoner's sentence plan, they are an integral part of the whole process. They have an important part to play in creating a climate conducive to addressing offending behaviour, dealing with drug misuse problems and preparing prisoners for release.

Model compacts

The main components of the model compact designed for use in all prisons and YOIs was set out by the Prison Service in 1993. The main features are as follows:

- a statement setting out the main elements of the standard regime;
- a statement detailing the extra privileges that apply to prisoners on the enhanced regime;
- the consequences of failing to abide by the terms of the compact, a statement explaining that a failure to keep to the terms of the compact is not in itself a disciplinary offence, unless the behaviour exhibited on a specific occasion constitutes a disciplinary offence;
- a statement that clarifies that the compact is an incentive and, whilst not compulsory, any prisoner who declines to sign a compact can only be offered the standard regime.

Compacts on a VTU

The compact on a VTU should be tailored to the specific needs of the unit. It should be discussed with the prisoner by the personal officer and the implications fully explained. The following issues should be comprehensively covered:

- the standards of behaviour expected on the wing, together with specific examples of behaviour that are clear breaches of the compact – e.g. possession of drugs, any drug use, or supplying drugs to others;
- the consequences of non-compliance;
- the avenues for raising a grievance or lodging an appeal against a decision made by the Incentives and Earned Privilege (IEP) Board;
- the process for reviewing the prisoner's care plan on the VTU.

The status of compacts

A compact is not a legal document; it is purely a voluntary agreement between the establishment and a prisoner and has no legal status. A prisoner cannot be compelled to sign a compact; he needs only to abide by its terms and conditions to receive the benefits it offers.

It is important to recognize that the IEP scheme and the prison discipline system are totally unrelated. This means that reducing a prisoner's privilege level (including removal from the VTU) must not be part of a disciplinary award because it would amount to double jeopardy.

However, proven disciplinary offences can affect a prisoner's privilege level if they amount to a pattern of behaviour and are brought to the attention of the monthly IEP Board.

Not surprisingly staff view very seriously certain offences, such as supplying or taking drugs whilst on a VTU. Following 'best practice' advice, issued from Prison Service headquarters, can avoid any possibility of double jeopardy and legal challenge

1. I agree to abstain completely from illegal drugs and alcohol.
2. I will not take part in any activity connected with the illegal use of drugs.
3. I agree to sign the 'Prisoner's Consent to the Transfer of Information' form allowing the CARAT worker to obtain confidential information about my medical and social background from other agencies.
4. I understand I am subject to the MDT programme in addition to the voluntary testing programme and that any positive MDT test will result in me being placed on Governor's report.
5. I realize that if I'm found guilty on adjudications of being in possession of any illegal substance, or fail an MDT, my privilege level will be reviewed and I risk losing my enhanced status.
6. I will cooperate with all routine searches and requests for voluntary random urine tests, and understand that a false or tampered reading will be deemed to be a positive test.
7. I will cooperate with drawing up a care plan and achieving agreed targets and will attend interviews, group meetings and drug awareness classes suggested by prison staff and CARAT workers.
8. I will not behave in an aggressive, threatening or violent manner, neither will I bully or intimidate others or use offensive language.
9. I will treat staff, visitors and other prisoners with respect irrespective of their race, ethnic origins, religious beliefs, gender, sexual orientation or social circumstances.
10. I will respect VTU policy on confidentiality, and understand that my privacy will be respected by staff, subject to the needs of security, child care and self-harm considerations being paramount.
11. I understand that no smoking, drinking or eating is allowed in group sessions or classes held on the VTU.
12. I will treat the wing and communal facilities with respect, and keep myself clean and tidy whilst resident on the unit.
13. I understand that all staff on the unit are committed to maintaining the unit drug-free and they will encourage all prisoners to address their drug problems by providing opportunities for personal counselling and attending groups and classes.
14. I understand as a voluntary member of the unit I can request a move to normal location at any time.

Signed . . . .   Signed . . . .
          (prisoner name and number)   (on behalf of the Governor)

Figure 8: The compact on a voluntary testing unit

arising. This advice suggests that the following condition should be included in all prisoner compacts: 'I am aware that should I be found guilty of being in possession of any controlled substance or failing a mandatory drugs test, my privilege level will be reviewed and I will be at risk of losing my enhanced status.'

The compact on a voluntary testing unit

This compact requires each prisoner to agree to the conditions shown in Figure 8 before they are allocated a place on the VTU. The compact is signed by the prisoner and by a member of wing staff on behalf of the Governor. One copy is given to the prisoner and another retained in the prisoner's case record.

INCENTIVES AND EARNED PRIVILEGES (IEP)

Every establishment has a local Incentives and Earned Privilege Scheme which conforms to the National Policy Framework and the Standards Manual. The main requirement is to state clearly and publicly how the system operates and to ensure that everyone has access to this information. The aims of the scheme are:

- to have in place a system of privileges which are earned as a direct result of good performance and behaviour, but which can be withdrawn if a prisoner fails to maintain an acceptable level of behaviour;
- to recognize and reward responsible behaviour;
- to encourage prisoners to work and use their time constructively;
- to help sentenced prisoners to progress through the prison system;
- to encourage prisoners to conform;
- to develop a better disciplined, more controlled and safer environment for staff and prisoners.

The scheme aims to encourage prisoners to cooperate whilst in custody. This is achievable if the scheme is just and is administered by fair, equitable and regular review procedure.

Since a review of the scheme in 1998, the level of private cash that prisoners can accumulate in their spending account has been restricted. The limit set is ten times the weekly limit applicable to the incentive schemes level.

Private cash restrictions do not apply to women in mother and baby units who can spend unlimited amounts of private cash on their babies or on pregnancy-related items. Overseas phone calls are exempt for anyone with close relatives abroad or who normally lives abroad, anyone involved in legal proceedings and any unconvicted prisoner who is continuing to keep a business running.

The underlying assumption of the IEP scheme is that every privilege above the basic level has to be earned. There are three levels of privilege: basic, standard and enhanced. These are separate to the minimum standards that apply to prisoners undergoing punishment in the segregation unit.

The published statement of facilities available to prisoners is reviewed on an annual basis. It sets out:

*   what privileges can be earned;
*   details of privileges that apply at each level and the criteria that must be met to earn and keep them;
*   how privileges are lost;
*   details of the procedures that are followed;
*   how the outcome of IEP reviews are communicated;
*   the correct way to make an appeal.

The basic regime

Convicted prisoners on the basic regime are restricted to the following:

*   *Private cash* – the allowance is £2.50 per week.
*   *Visits* – two half-hour visits every 28 days in the normal visits area.
*   *Association* – this is the time allowed out of a cell to take part in activities or associating with other prisoners, and is normally provided at a minimum level.

Prisoners on the basic regime do not qualify for community visits or the enhanced earnings scheme and cannot wear their own clothing.

An unconvicted prisoner on the basic regime is restricted to the following privileges:

*   *Private cash* – the allowance is £15 per week. This is higher than for convicted prisoners because unconvicted prisoners are not obliged to work.
*   *Visits* – a total of one and a half hours per week taken in the visits area.
*   *Association* – this provided at a fairly minimal level.
*   *Wearing own clothing* – an entitlement.

All prisoners on basic level must have their status reviewed at least monthly and young offenders reviewed every fourteen days.

Prisoners can avoid the basic regime by paying attention to the overall pattern of their institutional behaviour. The following issues need to receive particular attention:

*   How well do they conform to the routines and rules?
*   Are they regularly appearing on Governor's adjudications?
*   Do they get on with other prisoners?
*   How far do they cooperate with staff?
*   Do they attend educational classes or a training course?
*   Is their performance at work satisfactory?

Cooperating with, and becoming involved in, the sentence planning process is generally interpreted as a willingness to use the custodial experience constructively, as is forming a good relationship with the nominated personal officer. A prisoner's attitude towards outside contacts is monitored including the level, frequency and nature of contact with his own family, any contact with the victim, and the outside Probation Service.

The following may be included in local criteria for determining movement between the different levels of regime:

- *Non-violence* – an absence of aggression, threatening behaviour, bullying and the use of offensive language.
- *Non-discrimination* – an absence of racist, sexist, bigoted behaviour.
- *Civility* – considerate, polite behaviour.
- *Mutual respect* – cooperating with staff, complying with lawful requests and behaving openly and honestly.
- *Treatment of others* – developing supportive relationships with others.
- *Compliance with rules* – taking care of prison property and equipment, bending or breaking the regulations, drug-taking, substance abuse, gambling or bullying other prisoners.
- *Personal hygiene* – keeping himself and his cell clean and tidy.
- *Health and hygiene issues* – not posing a health hazard to others by using equipment recklessly, and adhering to fire precautions and smoking restrictions.
- *Achievements* – working industriously, attending training courses and offending behaviour groups and gaining recognized educational qualifications.

Cooperative prisoners are invariably placed on the standard regime.

The standard regime

Once staff are satisfied that a prisoner is unlikely to be problematic and has completed the induction phase satisfactorily, the prisoner is placed on the standard regime. The recommended level of key earnable privileges laid down in the national framework for convicted prisoners is as follows:

- *Private cash* – The allowance is £10.00 each week.
- *Visits* – At least three visits every 28 days, normally held in the visits area.
- *Association* – This corresponds to the norm for the establishment but is set at a higher level than for those on the basic regime.
- *Community visits* – Anyone allocated to a resettlement prison or wing is allowed a weekly community visit. Prisoners in an open prison, suitable young offenders or adult female prisoners are eligible for a monthly visit.
- *Enhanced earnings scheme* – Although eligible for consideration, priority is given to those on the enhanced regime.
- *Wearing own clothing* – Discretionary but uncommon for men; women can wear their own clothes if they are considered suitable.

An unconvicted prisoner on the standard regime can receive the following privileges:

- *Private cash* – The allowance is £30.00 each week.
- *Visits* – This varies between different types of establishment and is more frequent than for those on the basic regime.
- *Association* – This is at a higher level than the basic regime.
- *Enhanced earnings scheme* – Priority is given to those on the enhanced regime.
- *Wearing own clothing* – This is an entitlement.

The enhanced regime

Governors have considerable discretion to include additional privileges in their IEP Schemes. These can include any or all of the following:

- allocating the best jobs to those on the enhanced regime, such as work in the kitchen or 'red-bands' (positions of trust allocated to carefully vetted individuals);
- additional items of cell furniture above the laid-down minimum standard;
- the use of cooking facilities on the wing;
- dining in association;
- electronic games;
- additional sessions in the gymnasium;
- access to laundry facilities;
- additional opportunities to use the facilities in the library;
- purchasing items by mail order;
- flexibility regarding meal times within defined time bands;
- extra newspapers;
- having their own duvet as an alternative to prison bedding;
- in-cell television, using sets provided by the Prison Service at a weekly rental of £1 per set;
- any other permissible items such as having curtains, a bedspread, flask, rug or rechargeable batteries in their cell.

The Governor must ensure additional privileges do not contravene the volumetric control policy which requires the total amount of personal possessions to fit into two prison-issue boxes of a standard size.

The incentive for prisoners to conform and progress to the enhanced regime is considerable. The following privileges, laid down in the national framework, are recommended for convicted prisoners on the enhanced regime:

- *Private cash* – The allowance is £15.00 each week.
- *Visits* – The frequency is greater than on the standard regime and where possible four or five one-hour visits every 28 days are allowed. Flexibility exists regarding where these visits take place and the conditions that apply.
- *Association* – This can be up to twelve to fourteen hours daily.
- *Community visits* – Prisoners in a resettlement prison or wing are permitted one

every week; those in open conditions can have two visits each month; and other category D prisoners, selected young offenders and female prisoners qualify for one each month.

* *Enhanced earnings scheme* – They are eligible for this privilege.
* *Wearing own clothing* – This is permissible.

Unconvicted prisoners on the enhanced regime can receive the following privileges:

* *Private cash* – The allowance is £30.00 each week.
* *Visits* – This is set at a level higher than the standard regime, although the scope is reduced by the limited facilities and level of overcrowding that occurs in a local prison.
* *Association* – This is greater than the standard regime.
* *Enhanced earnings scheme* – This is unlikely to be possible.
* *Wearing own clothing* – This is an entitlement.

Local IEP Schemes should be integrated into sentence management and through-care arrangements. The IEP Scheme should take into account the views of the prisoner when reviewing privilege levels. The views of a range of staff should be obtained, with the personal officer and a senior manager involved in the decision-making.

Compacts on the voluntary testing unit should fully reflect the aims of the IEP Scheme. They should encourage prisoners to behave responsibly, work hard, become involved in constructive activity, and to address their offending behaviour and drug misuse problems.

CASE STUDY

John is discovered with a smoking device

During a routine cell search on the voluntary testing unit, a smoking device, similar to those used for 'chasing the dragon', is found hidden in his cell locker. John is charged under Prison Rule 51 paragraph 12, that he 'has in his possession any unauthorized article', namely a smoking device used for taking controlled drugs.

Although John admits the offences, he claims in mitigation that he no longer takes drugs and the smoking device belongs to another inmate. John claims he was only looking after the device for him. His conduct report reveals it is his first disciplinary offence, that he is normally well behaved and cooperates fully with staff. The Governor imposes the standard level of punishment for that type of offence and warns him that he is liable for an MDT test as he is not convinced by his explanation and believes he is using drugs. The Governor warns John that a positive test result would make him liable for further punishment.

John's problems are not over because he is in breach of the compact he signed when admitted to the VTU. He is given a final warning by the wing manager that another drug-related offence will result in removal from the VTU. In the meantime, his privilege level will be reviewed at the next monthly IEP Board, when he is at risk of losing his enhanced status.

Three weeks later, the IEP Board meet to review John's privilege level along with other prisoners in the wing; the board decides to downgrade him to standard level. The reasons for this decision are explained to John and they are his deteriorating attitude and overall standard of behaviour, as well as genuine concern that he is relapsing into drug misuse.

CHECKLIST

- What is a CARAT worker?
- For which prisoners does the CARAT process cater?
- How soon after initial contact should a full CARAT assessment be carried out?
- What is the purpose of the Prisoner's Consent to the Transfer of Information form?
- Does written consent for disclosure of confidential information extend to third parties?
- Who is involved in preparing the care plan?
- What are SMART targets?
- How is the CARAT release plan prepared?
- What is the role of the CARAT worker for prisoners discharged locally?
- How is support provided following release when the prisoner is discharged to a local address?
- Identify the aims of a voluntary testing unit.
- Why does the drug strategy unit recommend the use of dip and read testing?
- What are multiple screening tests?
- Identify the limitations of dip and read tests.
- Is it obligatory to have a prisoner compact in place on a VTU?
- How do compacts for prisoners on a VTU differ from those elsewhere in the establishment?
- What are the three levels of privilege under the Incentive and Earned Privilege Scheme?
- How often should the Incentive and Earned Privilege Board meet to review a prisoner's privilege level?
- In what ways does the published IEP Scheme encourage prisoners on a VTU to behave responsibly, use their time constructively and address their drug problems?

CHAPTER 7

Drug Treatment Programmes

THE HEALTH CARE STRATEGY

The corporate plan for the Prison Service reflects the Government's priorities of 'Protecting the Public' and 'Reducing Crime'.

A major objective of 'Reducing Crime' is, by 2002, to:

Improve the assessment, support and resettlement of drug misusing offenders and improve the availability and quality of drug treatment; reduce the supply of drugs into prisons; provide opportunities for prisoners to be located in voluntary testing units in order to remain free of drugs; and to establish the effectiveness of the drug strategy through evaluation and research.

Health care objectives

There are three major health care objectives in 'Protecting the Public'; by 2002 the Prison Service intends to:

1. Establish, with the NHS, a new Joint Prison Health Policy unit, responsible for the development of prison health policy, drawing on, and integrating with, wider national health policies. This new policy unit would replace the present Prison Service Directorate of Health Care.
2. Undertake joint work between health authorities and prison Governors to identify the health needs of prisoners in their area, and to develop Prison Health Improvement Programmes. This phase should be completed by 2000.
3. Establish a Joint Prison Health Care Task Force to help support prisons and health authorities, to drive forward the assessment of health needs, and the changes identified by the Prison Health Improvement Programmes.

    The planned series of health improvement programmes should commence during the period 2000–2.

A survey by the Office for National Statistics revealed a high incidence of mental ill health in the prison population. Approximately 90 per cent of all prisoners have one or more of the main types of mental disorder, which include psychosis, neurosis, personality disorder, alcohol misuse and drug dependence.

Supporting drug misusers

Taking drugs prescribed by a general practitioner or obtained from a pharmacist is not without risks. All legitimate drugs are thoroughly tested and their production is strictly licensed as they can have unpleasant side effects or an allergic reaction can occur. In addition, GPs take care to avoid prescribing combinations of certain drugs which can be harmful and react adversely if taken together.

Illegal drugs pose a serious risk to health because they are often contaminated with other substances, such as talcum powder or laxatives, and are often mixed with other drugs. This makes predicting the likely side effects an uncertain business, although it can be said for certain that they can be both unpleasant and dangerous. Injecting any contaminated drugs, particularly if the syringe or needle has not been sterilized, increases enormously the risk of contracting hepatitis, HIV and other blood-borne diseases.

The role of health care staff

Health care staff have a crucial role to play in making need assessments and treating drug misusers. They have a responsibility to examine and interview everyone on first reception.

Whilst it is appreciated that many of those with a drug problem are reluctant to admit as much, some prisoners are more willing to admit they have a drug problem in a medical environment. However, outside agencies have reported that as few as 10 per cent of prisoners reported their drug problems to the prison authorities prior to the introduction of CARAT services in establishments.

Health care staff must provide relevant information to prisoners about the range of help that is available in the establishment, refer them to relevant specialist services and provide appropriate medical care, including detoxification.

Developing an inter-disciplinary approach

The importance of developing an inter-disciplinary approach to tackling drug abuse in prison cannot be over-emphasized. As soon as prisoners are received into custody, trust needs to be established and relationships formed with the Probation Service, personal prison officers, education staff, the chaplain and prison psychologist. Some prisoners who are seeking help with a drug problem are concerned that disclosure may adversely affect their level of privileges or their chances of release under licence.

The importance of respecting prisoner confidentiality and handling drug dependency problems sensitively is of paramount importance if more prisoners are to be encouraged to seek help.

THE RISKS OF HIV/AIDS

The Human Immunodeficiency Virus (HIV) gradually but systematically destroys the immune system and is the virus that can cause AIDS. The HIV virus attacks the CD4 cell which enables the immune system to function properly. Once the CD4 cells have reduced over several years to a third of their original number, the immune system is unable to resist certain diseases and the individual gets ill through repeated infections. It is at this point they are described as having the Acquired Immune Deficiency Syndrome (AIDS).

The time-span from the first diagnosis of HIV to the development of AIDS varies considerably. Some develop the illness within two years but generally about 50 per cent of the infected HIV population have progressed to AIDS in ten years. Once AIDS is diagnosed, life expectancy can be as little as 20 to 30 months, although medical advances are extending this period. There is no vaccine available that offers protection against the HIV virus.

In 1997, out of a prison population in excess of 60,000, only 123 prisoners tested positive for HIV.

The HIV antibody test

Any prisoner who is concerned he might have the HIV virus can be tested and receive counselling. The test consists of an ordinary blood test which can be analysed for the presence of antibodies to HIV. Any antibodies detected mean the individual has the virus in their body and they are said to be HIV antibody positive, often shortened to HIV positive or body positive.

The problem with the test is that antibodies are produced three months after a person becomes infected with the virus. The period between becoming infected and the appearance of antibodies is known as the window period. During this time, a prisoner can be highly infectious yet produce a negative test. It is therefore important the test is conducted three months after the last occasion on which they could have become infected.

The risks to drug abusers

There are only three ways that the HIV virus can be spread to another person:

- *Unprotected sexual intercourse.*
  This normally occurs through unprotected vaginal or anal intercourse; although oral sex is less risky, it is not entirely safe.
- *From an infected mother to her baby.*
  A woman infected with HIV who becomes pregnant may infect her unborn baby in the womb, whilst giving birth or when breastfeeding. The likelihood of the virus being passed on to the unborn baby is 1:6, but treating the mother with antiviral drugs during pregnancy has further reduced the risks.
- *Blood spread.*
  Initially there was a risk of catching the virus from blood transfusions, and haemophiliacs were at high risk. This risk has been virtually eliminated since all blood donations are now tested for the virus. Now transmission of the virus

through blood can be almost entirely attributable to drug abusers sharing needles, and is the way HIV can spread amongst prisoners.

The main dangers facing prisoners are of unprotected sex and of using un-sterilized needles or syringes. These risks are emphasized in the updated educational videos available in every establishment called *AIDS Inside and Out* and *Talking About AIDS* and in a new information booklet *HIV and AIDS*, which is being issued to prisoners.

HEPATITIS AND OTHER COMMUNICABLE DISEASES

There are three different unrelated hepatitis viruses, A, B and C. Hepatitis A is the least serious. It is spread in contaminated water and food. Hepatitis B and C cause acute inflammation of the liver and can lead to serious liver diseases such as cirrhosis many years later. Hepatitis B and C are contagious and easily spread by infected blood or saliva getting into an open wound. The risks are very high in the prison environment if prisoners habitually share needles. Needle-stick injuries are particularly hazardous, as there is a high risk of infection if the needle contains blood from an infected carrier of hepatitis B.

Hepatitis B

It is estimated there are 300 million people worldwide who are seriously ill with this virus; this makes it more widespread than HIV. About 40 per cent of those who become affected develop acute hepatitis with jaundice after an incubation period of about two to six months; of that number about 1 in 100 die. The remaining 60 per cent experience few symptoms and invariably do not need medical attention, as they eventually develop antibodies and overcome the infection. A small proportion of these, about 6 per cent, become hepatitis carriers and this can last for the rest of their lives. They can also suffer serious liver disease and a few die from liver cancer.

Often those who become infected with the virus do not feel unwell and are often unaware they are affected. Fortunately, they cannot easily infect others unless they share needles or engage in unprotected sex. However, it can also be spread by urine, which is why care needs to be exercised by everyone involved in handling containers used for taking urine samples in the mandatory drug testing centre.

All prisoners and prison staff (including members of the BoV and others in regular contact with prisoners) are entitled to be vaccinated on request. A full course of the vaccine comprises three doses spread over six months which gives protection for three to five years against normal risks. It cannot offer protection against unprotected sex with an infected person, or protect drug injectors who share needles.

Hepatitis C

Hepatitis C is a relatively new virus which was identified in 1989. Although there are about 250,000 infected with this virus in the UK, there is no vaccine available, nor any prospect of one in the immediate future. It is easily transmitted by needle-sharing, by tattooing or by needle-stick injuries, particularly in the prison environment, where the equipment is unlikely to be sterilized. It is not readily transmitted by unprotected sexual activity, but can be passed from a mother to her baby in the womb, or when she is breastfeeding.

Some prisoners infected with hepatitis C develop acute hepatitis with jaundice, and can develop other symptoms such as arthritis and rashes. One problem is that antibodies can take up to a year to develop naturally to fight the virus. As many as 50–70 per cent of those infected develop a mild form of chronic hepatitis which continues indefinitely and does not heal. Over a lengthy period of time, ten to twenty years, this can develop into serious forms of liver disease such as cirrhosis.

Tuberculosis

Tuberculosis, commonly known as TB, is an infection caused by the germ *Mycobacterium tuberculosis*. It attacks the lungs, lymph nodes, kidneys, bones, joints and the membranes around the brain (known as meninges). Anyone infected with HIV is particularly susceptible to becoming infected with pulmonary tuberculosis, an infection of the lungs by tubercle bacilli.

Tuberculosis normally responds well to treatment by drugs. However, in some cases serious illness develops leading to eventual death, as the lungs and other organs are progressively destroyed by the bacterium.

Conditions which are conducive to the spread of tuberculosis are confined and poorly ventilated places. If an infected person coughs and sneezes, the infected droplets become airborne, easily spreading the disease in the prison environment.

The Bacillus Calmete-Guérin (BCG) vaccination is usually successful as it works by raising an individual's level of immunity. However, anyone whose immune system has been weakened by the HIV virus is extremely vulnerable to infection.

There is evidence in New York that the tubercle bacilli are becoming resistant to most of the drugs used to treat this illness. In the USA, where large numbers of HIV positive prisoners have been kept together, this has provided an opportunity for the disease to spread rapidly.

The tuberculin test is used to assess a person's immune system. Anyone who is tuberculin-negative has no resistance and must be vaccinated with BCG.

Prisoners who are susceptible to tuberculosis are those:

* who have been homeless;
* who come from a very deprived background;
* who are HIV positive;
* who have a history of misusing drugs;
* who have been living in Africa, Asia or Latin America prior to coming into custody.

ISSUING DISINFECTING TABLETS

Although the Prison Service policy on drugs unequivocally commits it to reducing the level of drug misuse in establishments, it has to balance this policy against its responsibility to help prisoners who misuse drugs. A significant number of prisoners who inject themselves with illegal drugs in the community continue the practice after they are received into custody. They tend to share needles and syringes, which puts their own health and safety at risk. It also exposes staff and other prisoners to needle-stick injuries which in turn increases the risk of transmitting HIV and hepatitis.

In 1999, a pilot project was initiated which makes available to prisoners and young offenders disinfecting tablets, together with information leaflets. There are eleven establishments taking part in this initiative: Norwich, Woodhill, Wealstun, Coldingley, Garth, Long Lartin, Cookham Wood, Askham Grange, Holloway, Highdown and Stoke Heath. The scheme may be extended to all establishments after the results have been evaluated. The disinfecting tablets used are similar to those used to sterilize babies' bottles; they are completely safe even if prisoners swallow them or attempt to burn them. If the tablets are burned, a very small amount of chlorine gas is released which immediately reacts with the air and forms a non-hazardous gas.

Controlling the spread of infection

Issuing disinfecting tablets is aimed at controlling the spread of HIV and other infectious diseases. It also enables prisoners determined to inject drugs to minimize the risks to themselves and others by using clean needles and syringes. Prisoners are being advised that this is a risk-reducing initiative and does not guarantee the possibility of transmitting viruses is completely eliminated.

The operating principles that apply with this scheme are twofold: to avoid drug injectors having to identify themselves; and to make disinfecting tablets readily accessible to users.

In Scotland, where this initiative was successfully introduced in 1993, the methodology adopted was to place tablets in common areas such as the kitchen, recesses and lavatories, where prisoners could obtain them unseen by staff.

This project is being independently assessed by a team from the London School of Hygiene and Tropical Medicine and their report and recommendations are currently under consideration.

HEALTH EDUCATION

Following publication of the report The Future Direction of Education Provision in HM Prisons, Young Offender Institutions and Remand Centres (1997), every establishment must offer the National Curriculum Framework of Core Skills. There are four main programmes: Communications, Numeracy, Information Technology, and Social and Life Skills.

The Social and Life Skills programme is designed to complement other courses that address offending behaviour, such as the Sex Offender Treatment Programme, the Enhanced Thinking Skills Programme, and the Reasoning and Rehabilitation Programme. Its purpose is to encourage prisoners to develop their personal awareness and social, personal and vocational skills. It aims to address prisoner needs as well as develop their self confidence and self esteem.

Social and Life Skills

The Social and Life Skills curriculum is offered as an accredited course at three different levels:

1. *Basic Skills Test in Life Skills*
   This is accredited by the Associated Examination Board and is suitable for young offenders.
2. *Social and Life Skills programme*
   This is accredited by the Open College Network and is suitable for all penal establishments.
3. *Diploma in Achievement*
   This is accredited by the Oxford and Cambridge Diploma in Achievement.

Accreditation means that every module that is successfully completed can have a credit awarded, which is equivalent to GCSE, NVQ and GNVQ.

The Social and Life Skills programme is offered at Levels 1 and 2. Each level comprises eleven units, which requires twenty hours of teacher contact time to complete to the required standard. The units available are:

- preparation for work;
- family relationships;
- parentcraft;
- working with others;
- budgeting and money management;
- cookery;
- do-it-yourself;
- healthy living;
- introduction to drug and alcohol awareness;
- improved assertiveness and decision-making;
- personal development.

Drug and Alcohol Awareness

This unit has five modules:

1. drugs and their misuse;
2. effects of misusing drugs;
3. short- and long-term effects of consuming alcohol;
4. alcohol abuse and its effects;
5. agencies offering help and support.

Those prisoners who complete the course are assessed against a set of explicit learning outcomes, and undertake assignments, exercises and short projects and they make presentations and take part in discussions.

The unit covering Drug and Alcohol Awareness covers the following issues:

1. *Drugs and their misuse*
    This module examines the physical risks and mental effects of drug misuse, and includes imparting knowledge about the main groups of drugs. Prisoners are advised about the particular dangers facing vulnerable groups, such as pregnant women and solvent abusers.
2. *Effects of misusing drugs*
    This module helps prisoners to appreciate the personal and social causes of drug abuse. It examines how drug abuse adversely affects personal relationships and the quality of their social life. The link between drug misuse and crime is explored and prisoners are encouraged to examine how drug dependency can affect their prospects in life.
3. *Short- and long-term effects of consuming alcohol*
    This module helps prisoners understand the physical risks and mental effects of alcohol use, and points out the possible damage alcohol abuse has on the body, such as cirrhosis of the liver.
4. *Alcohol abuse and its effects*
    This module helps promote understanding about the personal and social causes of alcohol abuse. It identifies the potential effects on family, friends, work colleagues and the individual's finances.
5. *Agencies offering help and support*
    This module identifies the agencies that offer information to drug users in the community. It highlights where help is available, which agencies and organizations exist, what they do, who they help and the level of support available.

DETOXIFICATION PROGRAMMES

Detoxification is the term used to describe the treatment process associated with getting rid of toxins (poisons) from the body. Detoxification treatment programmes need close medical supervision, and prisoners are normally admitted as inpatients to the prison hospital or special detoxification unit.

Some drugs, such as heroin, alcohol and tranquillizers, are physically addictive and the body experiences withdrawal symptoms if the availability of these drugs suddenly stops. These symptoms can vary from discomfort to pain. In some cases it is dangerous suddenly to stop taking a highly addictive drug, as the individual needs to be gradually weaned from drug dependence.

Drugs such as cocaine and amphetamines (speed) are not as physically addictive and prisoners can safely stop using them without the need for medical intervention.

The Prison Service policy is to offer detoxification to any prisoner who presents signs of addiction. These are verified following examination by a medical officer and confirmation by the prisoner's own GP. £10.8 m of CSR funding has been allocated to improving detoxification services in local prisons and remand centres in 1999–2000. The aim is to offer drug detoxification to 18,000 prisoners each year in accordance with the guidelines produced by the Prison Service Healthcare Standard 8. This is being revised to bring it into line with the latest NHS guidance and to provide prisoners with a service which is of equal quality to that available in the community.

Managing withdrawal from opiates

The problem facing opiate users is that heroin is very addictive and regular users develop a tolerance to the drug. This means they have to take a bigger dose to get the same effect and this results in physical dependence. Weaning regular users off heroin can produce unpleasant side effects, such as diarrhoea, nausea, vomiting, stomach cramps, muscle spasms, flu-like symptoms, depression, irritability, general moodiness, discomfort and pain.

Injecting heroin brings additional dangers of damaged veins and gangrene, in addition to the risks associated with sharing needles (HIV and hepatitis).

Detoxification programmes are normally available in local prisons and normally offered to new receptions who are addicted to opiates. Patients are admitted to the prison hospital where they receive a treatment programme consisting of decreasing doses of methadone (physeptone linctus) in liquid form, over a seven-day period.

A routine detoxification programme would take the following form, with the initial two-day period constituting an assessment period:

Day 1   Normally up to 40–50 mg of methadone linctus administered in smaller doses depending on the time of reception.

Day 2   30 mg of methadone linctus, with 10 mg administered in the morning (AM), during the afternoon (PM) and overnight (ON).

Day 3   25 mg of methadone linctus, with 10 mg AM, 5 mg PM, and 10 mg ON.

Day 4   20 mg of methadone linctus, with 10 mg AM and 10 mg ON.

Day 5   15 mg of methadone linctus, with 5 mg AM, 5 mg PM and 10 mg ON.

Day 6   10 mg methadone linctus, with 5 mg AM and 5 mg PM.

Day 7   5 mg methadone linctus administered AM.

In the case of pregnant women and AIDS patients, this treatment programme would be modified to ensure a more gradual reduction. Instead of cutting down the dosage by 5 mg per day, the reduction takes place over several weeks at the rate of 5 mg per week. A more extended withdrawal regime minimizes the physiological and emotional stress of the treatment and avoids the individual being tempted to seek relief from the withdrawal symptoms through illegal drug-taking.

Some medical officers may treat the side effects associated with the treatment with analgesics and antispasmodics, whilst the drug naltrexone (Nalorex) is sometimes used to combat the craving for opiates during treatment.

It is very important that, when using methadone treatment in custody, careful monitoring takes place when dispensing the prescribed drugs; there is a risk that, without adequate safeguards, methadone may find a way onto the black market in the establishment. All prisoners accepted on a methadone treatment programme should enter into a contract with the establishment and agree to have regular confidential voluntary urine tests; to have their treatment discontinued if they are found to be taking any non-prescribed drugs; and to remain liable to mandatory drug testing and consequent disciplinary action.

Detoxification at HMP Lindholme

At HMP Lindholme health care centre, an opiate detoxification programme exists in which the drug *lofexidine hydrochloride* (Britlofex) has been used successfully to combat withdrawal symptoms. This product is the first non-addictive and non-opiate drug on the market and is available in tablet form. Although it can cause hypertension, the drug has been shown to reduce withdrawal symptoms. It is suitable for self-administration and can be used safely in the penal environment and in the community.

The detoxification programme operating at Lindholme lasts for seven days and commences with the taking of a urine sample which is tested for opiates. Each day the prisoner undergoing the programme is given 0.2 mg tablets of lofexidine at 1000 hours in the health care centre and is given a further tablet to take at 1400 hours. At 1600 hours he returns to the health care centre for a further treatment under supervision and is given a tablet to take at 1800 hours. By day seven, the detoxification is complete and he returns on the eighth day to give a final urine sample which is screened for the presence of opiates.

The staff in the health care centre ensure the prisoner is aware of the following points which are incorporated into a detoxification contract:

- They must take the medication at the stated times.
- They must not exceed the prescribed dosage.
- They must not take the medication more frequently than prescribed.
- They are aware of the possible side effects from taking this medication.
- They are aware of what action to take if they experience any side effects.
- They understand that under no circumstances will any medication given for the purpose of self-administration be replaced if lost or stolen.
- They can withdraw from the treatment programme at any time.
- In accordance with the Misuse of Drugs Regulations 1973, they will be notified to the Home Office addiction register.
- They agree to absolve the medical and health care centre staff from any responsibility for any adverse consequences if they deviate from the detoxification programme, and appreciate the programme may be terminated if they fail to comply with the detoxification contract.

Two encouraging features of the Lindholme approach, which is being emulated in other establishments, is that prisoners are taking some responsibility for the success of their own treatment and that this approach to opiate detoxification does not require admission to the prison hospital and means more prisoners who need help can receive it.

Managing withdrawal from other substances

Serious abuses of sedatives, such as benzodiazepines and barbiturates, need to be treated with care and a programme of withdrawal phased over a minimum period of four weeks. Care must be taken to ensure benzodiazepines are not abruptly withdrawn, as this exposes abusers to the risk of convulsions.

Prisoners who are polydrug abusers (those who abuse several drugs at the same time) may need to receive this treatment in conjunction with opiate detoxification.

Withdrawing from stimulants such as amphetamines and cocaine can lead to depression and paranoia. This may necessitate psychiatric help and treatment by antidepressants and tranquillizers.

Alcohol dependence can be treated with reducing doses of tranquillizers and multivitamin supplements. The potential side effects can be critical and include delirium tremens and seizures.

Auricular Acupuncture

Ear acupuncture has been developed to help prisoners who need to detoxify from stimulants such as cocaine, crack and amphetamines. This is a completely safe form of treatment which involves trained therapists inserting about five small sterile needles around each ear. Auricular acupuncture is designed to harmonize the body's energy flow and help get rid of body toxins. Such treatment is often used in conjunction with group therapy and counselling and helps relieve stress and prevent sleepless nights.

DRUG COUNSELLING

Health education alone does not persuade people to alter their behaviour. In the past, campaigns that alert prisoners to the dangers of intravenous drug use have not been particularly effective in persuading people to stop injecting drugs. A comprehensive treatment strategy should include:

- drug awareness classes;
- health education;
- groupwork;
- counselling aimed at supporting individuals and changing their behaviour.

It is very difficult to achieve the necessary level of motivation to stop drug-taking without support and encouragement. The drug user may be faced with physical, psychological and social problems which need tackling if they are to manage their drug dependency successfully.

The process of withdrawing from drugs or changing to a less harmful pattern of drug use is made more difficult because of the following:

- Some drugs are physically very addictive.
- Many users are psychologically dependent on the drugs they take.

- The act of taking drugs brings immediate relief, whereas the risks appear to be distant and minimal.
- The drug culture exerts a powerful influence, especially when family and friends are taking drugs.
- The lifestyle adopted by some users to sustain their drug habit when living in the community gives them a sense of purpose. If unemployed, their time is spent obtaining funds and making drug deals.

The aims of drug counselling

The main purpose of drug counselling is to help individuals identify, overcome or come to terms with their psychological problems, and manage social problems associated with drug-taking. Helping prisoners change their behaviour involves offering encouragement, the necessary motivation and sustaining them when the going gets tough. For some, this can involve assessing their needs and referring them to an appropriate treatment programme for help. Others, unable to stop altogether, may respond to a harm-reduction approach, when they learn to appreciate the harm they are doing to themselves and others.

A successful outcome would be persuading the prisoner to agree to reduce their intake of drugs, use only clean equipment and avoid sharing needles or syringes. Ongoing counselling support should focus on helping them maintain their motivation to keep off drugs and resist falling into temptation. Helping those on a harm-reduction programme is geared to encouraging them to persevere and not back-slide.

Making the break from drug dependency can be very difficult and presents individuals with significant psychological and social problems.

How counselling works

Counselling means having a series of interviews or counselling sessions to identify, confront and attempt to resolve the problems together. Several stages are involved:

1. establishing a confidential working relationship;
2. helping the prisoner to explain the problem and clarifying the issues involved;
3. reducing the problem to manageable proportions that can be tackled in a systematic way;
4. identifying the resources available to tackle the problem:
   (a) inner resources,
   (b) the extended family,
   (c) friends,
   (d) community-based groups;
5. deciding on a plan of action that can be realistically achieved together;
6. arranging a follow-up meeting, or series of counselling sessions.

Counsellors have to work within the constraints of a penal setting and take into account cultural pressures (within the prison and external environment), which encourage continual drug misuse. Their role is to help the individual appreciate the consequences to themselves and others of continuing drug misuse, by gaining insight into their patterns of behaviour and coping methods.

The benefits of counselling

The positive outcomes from a series of counselling sessions are:

- a greater awareness of the risks of drug-taking;
- a greater resolve to look after their health;
- a concern not to jeopardize the health of others;
- a desire to minimize the impact drugs have on their lives.

Other benefits include a greater awareness of what help is available in custody; where help can be obtained after release; and an appreciation of whether friends and family are likely to be supportive.

Individuals who undertake counselling usually benefit considerably and develop greater self-determination; increased self-confidence; improved relationships with family and friends; and an enhanced quality of life.

Counselling must be coupled with ongoing support in order to be effective. Drug education messages need to be made personal and pertinent to the individual if they are to have any kind of impact.

Types of counselling

The first priority is to create a climate of trust, then help the individual to feel secure and understood. By encouraging him to define the problem and suggest realistic and achievable goals, the drug user can acquire the necessary self-confidence to make lifestyle changes.

There are three main types of counselling available:

1. *Crisis-intervention counselling*
   This is when a major life event occurs and the drug user feels overwhelmed or highly stressed. Examples of this are:
   (a) being detained by police,
   (b) receiving a custodial sentence,
   (c) being diagnosed with HIV,
   (d) becoming separated from a partner or spouse,
   (e) having a child taken into care,
   (f) on the death of a family member due to a drug overdose.
2. *Decision-making counselling*
   This means having to decide whether to confront the drug-taking habit. It can be prompted by a life crisis or result from being challenged at a drug awareness class or drug treatment group.

3. *Problem-solving counselling*
    An individual may need advice and support in living with the repercussions that
    follow from making a decision to reduce his intake of drugs or follow a harm-
    reduction programme. These can include:
    (a) how to keep away from drugs in prison,
    (b) how to avoid sharing needles or equipment,
    (c) how to live with a partner on release who is a user,
    (d) how to avoid returning to the drug scene after discharge,
    (e) how to replace drugs in his life.

Ingredients for successful counselling

Drug counselling can only succeed with prisoners if the following criteria are fulfilled:

*   *accessibility* – the service must be accessible to prisoners;
*   *confidentiality* – the counsellor must earn trust by treating everything they are told
    in confidence;
*   *credibility* – the counsellor must have professional expertise and integrity;
*   *knowledge* – the counsellor must have a sound understanding of drugs and their
    effects coupled with an understanding of how drug users behave;
*   *attitude* – the counsellor must be neutral and have a non-judgemental approach;
*   *acceptance* – the counsellor must be open and fair, treating everyone equally,
    irrespective of their race, gender or background;
*   *time* – the counsellor must allow sufficient time to deal with the prisoner's problem
    thoroughly;
*   *professional competence* – a basic level of training in counselling is essential;
*   *ongoing support* – counselling is stressful and ongoing supervision, support and
    training must be provided to counsellors if they are to function effectively.

Deciding to give up drugs or change to a less harmful pattern of drug use can be a
major struggle which affects their family, friends and lifestyle. *Counselling is not a
panacea.* However, in the context of an integrated programme of treatment and
education, counselling has an important part to play, as it enables prisoners to make
necessary adjustments in a supportive environment.

DRUGS AND PSYCHIATRIC DISORDERS

Coping with imprisonment can be very difficult. It is not surprising that some
prisoners are tempted to turn to drugs for short-term relief. The obvious dangers of
giving way to temptation are that the individual can become ensnared in the drug
culture, leading to financial stress, emotional pressure and physical threats from the
drug barons.

Some research suggests there are other dangers, namely a link between drug use
and psychiatric disorders. There are three schools of thought. First, the casual link,

which is an unproven link between drug-taking and childhood experiences. Second, coincidental disorders – the likelihood that drug dependency and psychiatric disorders found in the same patients are entirely coincidental. And third, cause and effect, when there is a clear link between drug-taking and psychiatric disorders.

The casual link

Some researchers in the USA believe that there is a link between childhood experiences and the onset of drug dependency later in adult life. The theory is that social problems experienced as a child adversely affect the individual's personal development and susceptibility to drug dependence. The researchers believe a child suffering with anxiety states or a depressive disorder may, as he grows older, experiment with drugs or become over-reliant on medications.

These researches found that a small number of cocaine addicts who suffered with Attention Deficit Disorder (ADD) supported the hypothesis of a casual link between drug use and psychiatric disorders.

Coincidental disorders

Another view is that physical and psychiatric disorders occur independently of problems associated with drug dependency. Current medical advice is to maintain clinical vigilance, be sceptical and adopt a neutral stance in the absence of conclusive evidence to the contrary. Although symptoms of a recognizable psychiatric condition may be present, this can be purely coincidental and simply an additional problem requiring treatment.

Cause and effect

Misusing some controlled drugs can trigger psychiatric problems. Medical officers are well aware that taking amphetamines and cocaine can cause short-term psychotic episodes. Drug-dependent prisoners who stop taking drugs can experience withdrawal symptoms which are symptomatic of a psychiatric disorder. A depressive reaction is often experienced when someone initially stops taking amphetamines and cocaine. This can develop into clinical depression after a lengthy period of trying to withdraw from these drugs.

When an individual turns to drugs as a way of coping with a major life crisis, the trauma of the drug withdrawal process can reactivate the original anxiety state or depression. Under these circumstances professional help is necessary to treat the original psychiatric problem.

Some individuals find drug-taking can trigger a reoccurrence of a psychiatric condition that was previously treated successfully. Prisoners suffering from schizophrenia and depression are particularly vulnerable to a relapse if they resume taking cannabis.

TREATMENT PROGRAMMES

There is a range of treatment, counselling and support services, of differing levels of intensity, that is available to prisoners. However, most treatment programmes are over-subscribed.

Educational programmes and self-help support programmes are suitable for anyone who does not have a serious drug dependency problem.

A series of in-depth counselling sessions, which can be continued after release, may be more appropriate for those needing throughcare and treatment after release.

Modular-based programmes geared to the needs of those serving sentences of over six months usually require prisoners to attend for one to two days a week. These programmes may be provided on dedicated drug wings or voluntary testing units with support provided from the CARAT service provider.

Therapeutic communities

Therapeutic communities are provided in a few establishments and cater for the needs of those with behavioural and addiction problems. These regimes are more demanding than most prisoners expect because they require conformation with an agreed compact and full acceptance of responsibility for their behaviour.

The treatment involves expressing and dealing with feelings. This can be difficult and painful for some individuals, especially if they have spent all their life blaming others for their problems and avoiding responsibility for their actions.

HMP Grendon is a therapeutic prison that has wholeheartedly embraced the therapeutic community approach. All prisoners accepted for treatment take responsibility for supporting each other. Skilled help is available from medical officers, psychologists and specially trained discipline officers.

The Prison Service is committed to increasing the number of therapeutic communities, which it sees as a national resource. These dedicated residential units run intensive programmes for at least six months but more normally up to nine to twelve months. Currently, there are eight drug therapeutic communities, two of which cater for women.

Bail information and support

Prisoners are particularly vulnerable when they are first received into custody and need positive advice and guidance on reception. Those remanded in custody and charged with an offence that is unlikely to result in a custodial sentence can be considered for bail to a treatment facility. Initially, they are risk assessed to gauge their suitability then, providing they are acceptable and a suitable place can be found, they are taken onto the treatment programme. Once arranged, the court can be asked to approve the placement and grant bail.

This bail support service is normally organized by the Probation Service in conjunction with community-based drug agencies.

The twelve steps programmes

The twelve steps programme, known as the Minnesota Model on which it is based, was originally founded on the 'twelve steps to recovery' approach developed by Alcoholics Anonymous. This works on the assumption that addiction is a lifetime illness which can be controlled but never completely cured. Each step in the programme addresses a specific problem in the individual's life. He can move onto the next step only when the problem is resolved. It normally takes prisoners approximately three months to complete the twelve steps programme.

Individual counselling, groupwork and self-help groups are used and many of those involved in the treatment process are former addicts.

Self-help groups

The principle behind self-help groups is simply that prisoners with a common problem meet on a regular basis to offer each other support and encouragement. They have the advantage of having first-hand experience of the problem and can offer support at critical times – when the possibility of relapse is greatest.

Apart from Alcoholics Anonymous and Gamblers Anonymous, the main groups involved with support to drug users are Cocaine Anonymous and Narcotics Anonymous.

THE CHANNINGS WOOD EXPERIENCE

The New Directions Drug Therapeutic Community began as a pilot project and has been operating at HMP Channings Wood since 1997. It is run as a partnership between the establishment and the national charity Addaction. There is a twelve-month drug-free programme for adult, male, category C prisoners, based on a behavioural model used successfully at several prisons in the USA.

The therapeutic community occupies one wing in the prison and is run by twelve specially trained prison officers working alongside seven professional drugs workers from Addaction. The unit has 112 beds, of which 84 are for prisoners currently living in the therapeutic community; the remainder are reserved for those who, having successfully completed the programme, wish to continue living in a drug-free environment.

The Therapeutic Community compact

The New Directions Drug Therapeutic Community is a national resource and accepts referrals from throughout the country. The eligibility criteria is 'prisoners who are drug users with behavioural problems, willing to agree to enter into a compact to address their drug misuse problems'. The prisoner compact includes:

- cooperating fully with voluntary testing;
- understanding they will also be selected for mandatory drug tests;

- avoiding the use of any violence;
- no threatening or intimidatory behaviour;
- desisting from involvement with drug misuse.

Maintaining a drug-free environment depends largely on the ability of the therapeutic community to police and impose sanctions on residents who breach the rules. The residents decide collectively what penalties to impose for non-compliance, including the power to expel a member from the community.

Three positive drug tests, either as a result of voluntary or mandatory drug testing, normally result in expulsion from the community and a return to the sending establishment.

The treatment programme

This has three phases: orientation, primary treatment and re-entry. The programme length is variable because it responds to the individual's identified needs and capacity to progress through each stage of the treatment process.

1. *Orientation*
   The orientation phase, Induction and Training, lasts eight weeks. During this period the needs of prisoners are carefully assessed, education is provided, and the programme and rules explained.

2. *Primary Treatment*
   The second stage, Responsibility and Therapy, lasts between 16 and 24 weeks, and focuses on strategies that achieve positive and lasting behavioural change. It uses confrontation and encounter groups, which involve other residents pointing out how an individual's poor behaviour adversely affects others in the community. These groups are carefully supervised by staff who ensure it is the behaviour being confronted and not the individual.

3. *Re-entry*
   The final phase, Independence and Duty, lasts between twelve and sixteen weeks. It concentrates on re-integrating the individual into the community and facilitating support from community-based agencies.

The essence of the therapeutic approach is to agree personal goals with the prisoner. A personal key worker is assigned to work with them towards achieving these goals, which are then incorporated into a care plan.

The care plan is linked to the sentence management process and involves holding a sentence management review and devising a throughcare plan which prepares the prisoner for release.

The Incentive and Earned Privileges Scheme is linked to the treatment programme. Decisions about who holds positions of responsibility on the wing and their entitlement to receive additional privileges is dependent on each prisoner completing each of the three phases of the programme.

THE GROUPWORK APPROACH

Groupwork is a tried and tested approach which helps address offending behaviour. It enables learning to take place in a supportive setting alongside others facing similar problems.

Some learning techniques, such as role-play, can only be used in a group setting. Role-play allows an individual to rehearse his likely response in a given situation using video recordings and feedback from other members of the group.

An effective groupwork programme needs to incorporate the following:

- have a cognitive-behavioural approach which tries to change the way individuals react by helping them appreciate the connection between the way they think and the way they behave;
- be firmly structured;
- be multi-modal, tackling the whole range of problems they are facing at the same time;
- be based on a conceptual model with a sound theoretical understanding of the behaviour it is trying to change;
- be needs-based by demonstrating an appreciation of the individual's needs;
- be responsivity-orientated using techniques such as role-play and modelling which are known to be effective;
- have clearly defined targets;
- involve outside agencies;
- avoid eroding conditions such as returning those who complete a drug treatment programme to a wing which contains drug users;
- provide support to group leaders;
- be regularly reviewed and independently evaluated to make certain the agreed aims and objectives are being achieved.

Cognitive skills programmes

Cognitive skills training programmes address the thinking and reasoning processes which result in impulsive behaviour and also help prisoners who are having difficulty resolving conflict. The two programmes currently in use are:

1. *The Reasoning and Rehabilitation programme*
    This was imported from the Canadian Correctional Service and its syllabus includes:
    (a) values enhancement,
    (b) problem-solving skills,
    (c) creative thinking,
    (d) critical thinking,
    (e) interpersonal skills,
    (f) managing the emotional side of life.

2. *The Thinking Skills programme* covers:
   (a) impulse control,
   (b) rigid thinking,
   (c) creative thinking,
   (d) problem-solving,
   (e) perspective-taking,
   (f) decision-making.

Cognitive skills programmes help individuals develop new ways of thinking and reacting to problems and situations. They are particularly effective in helping drug misusers avoid relapse and gain understanding about social situations that they have difficulty handling appropriately.

PRE-RELEASE COURSES

Inmate development and pre-release courses are designed to help inmates cope with imprisonment and enable them to resettle successfully into the community on release. The course content is particularly relevant to helping drug misusers prepare for the challenge of release.

These courses encourage individuals to build their confidence and self-esteem, modify a poor attitude and realize their potential. They can learn new skills, heighten sensitivity towards others and gain practical advice about finding work, seeking accommodation, claiming benefits and health care matters. There are eleven modules in the complete course and these are the following:

1. *The communications package* which helps improve communication skills and encourages a greater awareness of the needs of others.
2. *The relationship package* which promotes self-awareness and assists individuals tackle relationship difficulties.
3. *The problem-drinking package* which increases knowledge about the negative effects of alcohol.
4. *The drugs package* which increases awareness about the risks associated with illicit drug-taking.
5. *The gambling package* which examines the risks and problems gambling can cause.
6. *The accommodation package* which assists individuals develop strategies for finding suitable accommodation.
7. *The money matters package* which helps them budget effectively and avoid the dangers of getting into debt.
8. *The standing-up-for-your-rights package* which explains how to exercise consumer and civil rights.
9. *The practical information package* which imparts information about DIY home maintenance, energy conservation, environmental issues, health care matters, survival cooking and using public transport.

10. *The work subject package* which focuses on providing information and advice which will help inmates re-enter the world of work.
11. *The time-on-your-hands package* which encourages the wise use of leisure time and examines ways of tackling problems facing the unemployed.

The multi-disciplinary nature of the inmate development and pre-release course means prison officers, teachers, probation officers, psychologists, chaplains, Physical Education Instructors (PEIs) and health care staff can all be involved in delivering parts of the programme. The course is in modular form, so those parts relevant to any identified needs can be incorporated into the sentence plan at the induction stage.

All these courses complement the throughcare approach introduced in the Criminal Justice Act 1991 and provide the opportunity to learn a range of skills that are useful in custody and designed to reduce the likelihood of reoffending.

CASE STUDY

John is concerned about HIV/AIDS

John's behaviour is causing great concern to his prison-based CARAT drug worker. He has recently been found guilty of having a smoking device in his cell, been downgraded to the standard level of privileges and his overall behaviour is poor.

His drug worker is convinced John has relapsed and his suspicions are borne out by a carefully supervised voluntary test conducted on the VTU, which gives a positive indication. John admits to avoiding testing positive on previous voluntary tests by cleverly adulterating his urine sample. He finally admits he has relapsed and has been sharing a needle with another prisoner. John admits he is worried about the risks he has been taking of contracting HIV/AIDS. He is referred to the medical officer who arranges for John to have an immediate HIV test, for the needle sharing and use of an unsterilized needle occurred more than three months ago. The test results indicate that he is not HIV positive, but John now appreciates he has taken serious risks and this is enough to convince himself that he needs further help.

He is admitted to the prison hospital to undergo further detoxification treatment which is accompanied by intensive drug counselling. He agrees to cooperate fully with his drug counsellor, and tries auricular acupuncture in an attempt to regain his motivation and the self confidence to rid himself of this habit.

As John is due for release in a few weeks' time, a place is organized for him on a pre-release course. In addition, the CARAT worker and probation officer focus on providing John and his family with effective post-release support from the local health authority and a community drug agency in his home area.

CHECKLIST

- Identify the three main health care objectives contained in the corporate plan for the Prison Service (1999–2002).
- How does the human immunodeficiency virus (HIV) develop into AIDS?
- Identify three ways the HIV virus can be spread throughout a prison.
- How are hepatitis B and C easily spread in the prison environment?
- Why are prisoners who have the HIV virus susceptible to infection with tuberculosis?
- How can the issuing of disinfecting tablets control the spread of infection?
- How do Social and Life Skills classes complement programmes that address offending behaviour?
- Describe the five components of the Drug and Alcohol Awareness unit offered under the Social and Life Skills curriculum.
- What is a detoxification programme?
- Why is it important for prisoners on a methadone treatment programme to enter into a contract with the establishment?
- How can polydrug abusers be treated?
- What is auricular acupuncture?
- How is drug counselling helpful to drug abusers?
- What are the aims of drug counselling?
- Describe how drug counselling works.
- Explain the differences between crisis-intervention counselling, decision-making counselling and problem-solving counselling.
- Is there an established link between drugs and psychiatric disorders?
- How does a therapeutic community help those with addiction problems?
- What is the Minnesota Model and how does it work?
- Describe the principles behind self-help groups.
- What are the components of an effective groupwork approach?
- Why can role-play be effective in a group setting?
- How does the Thinking Skills programme help those with drug misuse problems?
- What other cognitive skills programmes are available and how do they help prisoners?
- How do inmate development and pre-release courses prepare drug misusers for release?
- Why is a multi-disciplinary approach essential to helping those with drug problems?

CHAPTER 8

What Works?

TREATMENT WORKS

The limited research that has been done on the effectiveness of treatment and rehabilitation programmes in prisons strongly indicates that treatment is cost-effective, that drug use in prison is reduced and that fewer drugs are used after discharge.

A study in 1992 at Osteraker Prison in Sweden reveals that those who completed their eighteen-month drug treatment programme were 26.7 per cent less likely to relapse and return to custody than a control group at the same prison.

In the Netherlands it has been found that therapeutic drug-free units reduce the level of drug use in prisons and increase the likelihood of prisoners seeking treatment on release.

In Austria, Spain and the USA, methadone maintenance programmes have helped to reduce the number of prisoners sharing injecting equipment, and has made more prisoners predisposed to seek treatment on release.

HMP Downview

HMP Downview was the first establishment in this country to pilot drug treatment programmes in partnership with the Rehabilitation for Addicted Prisoners Trust (RAPt). The majority of prisoners admitted to their programme had a long-standing drug problem and attributed most of their criminality to drug dependency.

RAPt provide a twelve-step substance abuse treatment programme. This is based on total abstinence and offers aftercare to prisoners, thus assisting them to lead law-abiding lives on release. The programme is particularly effective because it is combined with comprehensive drug testing. At Downview they had a drug-testing machine, the SYVA ETS supplied by Behring.

The approach adopted at HMP Downview is as follows:

- on arrival prisoners are drug tested;
- any prisoner who tests positive on three occasions is transferred out;
- all prisoners undergo a three-month-long rehabilitation programme, run in partnership with the team from RAPt;

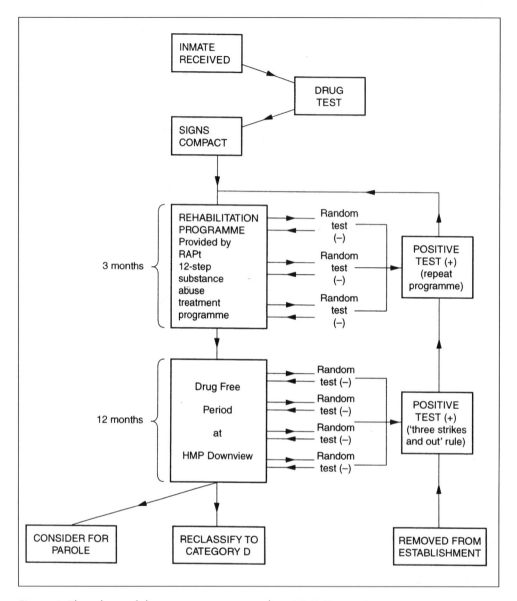

Figure 9: Flowchart of the treatment approach at HMP Downview

- a positive drug test whilst on the programme means having to repeat the twelve-step treatment programme;
- there is considerable peer group pressure to keep the prison drug-free.

Since drug programmes commenced at HMP Downview, there has been a significant reduction in drug use, as a sample of 23 prisoners showed. Ninety per cent of all those who successfully completed the programme remained drug-free. This conclusion was supported by the results of random drug testing.

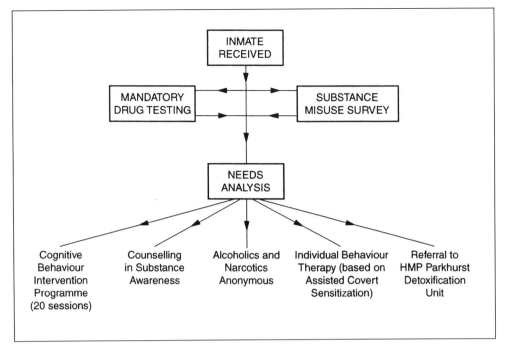

Figure 10: Flowchart of the treatment approach adopted at HMP Albany

Over a four-year period, the number of positive voluntary drug tests has fallen consistently. In 1994, there were 1413 positive results; in 1995, 1190 positive results; 1996, 461 positive results and in 1997, 416 positive results. By 1997–8, the number of positive voluntary drug tests had fallen to 4 per cent, suggesting that as many as 96 per cent of all prisoners are drug-free.

Crime and drug misuse

The link between crime and drug misuse has been clearly established through research. The National Treatment Outcome Research Study, funded by the Department of Health, found 70,000 crimes were committed by 1100 drugs misusers in the three months before they commenced drug treatment programmes.

A recent study in Leicester of 148 persistent drug offenders found that 42 per cent of them received a prison sentence on conviction.

Once admitted to prison or YOI, 10 per cent of male prisoners and 25 per cent of female prisoners were found to be drug-dependent.

Community-based studies

Some treatment programmes in the USA have proved very successful. Therapeutic communities, methadone maintenance programmes and community-based drug-free programmes can all lead to measurable reductions in illegal drug use.

The National Treatment Improvement Evaluation Study conducted in the USA in 1996 found that those completing treatment programmes were able to reduce their drug use significantly in the year following their attendance on the treatment programme. The main findings were that half the participants reduced their drug use and the level of arrests for offending fell by two thirds.

The Department of Health in the UK commissioned the National Treatment Outcome Research Study in 1995. This evaluated a range of drug treatment programmes. Almost all of the 1100 sampled were polydrug users, with the vast majority being long-term heroin users. The sample found that 37 per cent were using benzodiazepines regularly and 16 per cent were regularly using crack cocaine.

The effect on those attending drug treatment programmes has been significant and positive:

- *Residential programmes*
  Heroin use stopped completely within a month of the programme commencing.
- *Methadone maintenance programmes*
  Heroin use fell by 43 per cent.
- *Methadone reduction programmes*
  Heroin use fell by 61 per cent.
- *In-patient treatment units*
  Heroin use fell by 40 per cent.

The researchers report that similar levels of improvement with other drugs was recorded.

Community drug treatment services

One difficulty facing those seeking community-based drug treatment and rehabilitation services is the length of waiting lists. The Department of Health set up a task force to review services for drug users in November 1995. They found 64 per cent of residential services and 61 per cent of drug dependency clinics had waiting lists. The task force stresses the importance of drug users being able to gain access to treatment services on demand, for the following reasons:

- drug users are a vulnerable group;
- their motivation has to be channelled constructively because it is usually short-lived;
- the risks of harming themselves through continuing to misuse drugs are high.

The task force reached three clear conclusions following their review of services for drug misusers:

1. drug misuse is a chronic relapsing condition;
2. at least one attempt at treatment is necessary;
3. the longer the treatment continues the greater the chances of success.

In November 1995, the Standing Conference on Drug Abuse (SCODA), now Drug Scope, approached 124 drug agencies and found that a shortage of funding was making it more difficult for those in need to gain access to drug services. Some local authorities are unwilling to assess prisoners before discharge which denies them the opportunity to receive an appropriate level of throughcare. This reluctance to become involved before release is because prisoners may not serve their sentence in an establishment that lies within the boundaries of the local authority in which they normally reside.

This problem can be addressed in a variety of ways:

- providing adequate funding for drug aftercare services throughout the country;
- providing aftercare for drug misusers on a national basis;
- making local authorities financially responsible for the throughcare of prisoners who normally reside in their area until after their release;
- ensuring prisoners with drug dependency problems are returned to establishments in their home area prior to release;
- providing more resettlement prisons throughout the prison estate which have comprehensive drug treatment facilities and voluntary testing units.

The difficulties facing the Prison Service are unlikely to ease in the short term. The prison population in August 2000 was 66,141 and on current projections is likely to rise still further.

EVALUATING DRUG TREATMENT PROGRAMMES

The Prison Service piloted 21 drug treatment and rehabilitation programmes in nineteen establishments between 1995 and 1997.

PDM Consulting Ltd were asked by the Prison Service Directorate of Health Care to evaluate these pilot projects and make recommendations that develop the Prison Service strategy to extend drug treatment programmes. They produced their final report in February 1998: Evaluation of Prison Drug Treatment and Rehabilitation Services. It contains sixteen recommendations aimed at helping the Prison Service achieve its stated goal 'to achieve access by all establishments to a comprehensive range of prevention, treatment and rehabilitation programmes which meet the needs of all prisoners: those that have misused drugs and those that have not'.

Summary of recommendations

The recommendations contained in the report are as follows:

1. *Strategic Direction*
   Extend the pilot programmes so examples of good practice are made available to all prisoners.

2. *Inter-Agency Partnerships*
   Develop joint working arrangements with the National Health Service, Probation Service, social services and other public and voluntary agencies to ensure effective throughcare is offered to those attending drug treatment programmes.
3. *Coordinated Networks*
   Develop a coordinated approach based on the existing geographical structure, with an Area Drugs Coordinator to disseminate good practice and ensure minimum standards across the area. This is particularly important with women's and young offender establishments.
4. *Improving Drug Treatment*
   Aim to develop continually existing drug treatment programmes and seek to incorporate best practice into future programmes.
5. *Improving Programme Design*
   Improve the design of programmes by ensuring standardized assessment procedures are followed. This should cover guidance on voluntary drug testing, the intensity of treatment offered, medical prescribing practice and prisoner compacts.
6. *Women, Young Offender and other Specialist Populations*
   Programmes need to cater for the specialist needs of women, vulnerable prisoners, young offenders and prisoners in the dispersal system.
7. *Marketing and Promotion*
   Promote drug treatment programmes and target those most likely to benefit from them. Link the programmes offered to the Incentive and Earned Privilege System (IEPS), ensuring that the limited number of places are targeted at highly motivated, mature prisoners who are certain to benefit. Such prisoners make good ambassadors for drug treatment programmes.
8. *Use of Specialist Support*
   Ensure specialist NHS services are used wherever possible for detoxification and specialist supervision after release.
9. *Basic and Enhanced Services*
   Develop a range of services based on the assessed needs of selected prisoners which are sufficiently intense and geared to the amount of time they have to serve before release.
10. *Prisoners who are not Drug Users*
    Provide access to drug-free units for prisoners who don't use drugs and encourage them to remain drug-free.
11. *Internal Communication*
    Improve internal communications by involving staff and prisoners before introducing new programmes.
12. *Staff Selection*
    Identify well motivated staff who have the necessary core competencies and interpersonal skills to support drug treatment programmes.
13. *Contracting and Service Level Agreements*
    Base all future programmes on service level agreements (SLAs) which incorporate agreed performance targets.

14. *Financial Management*
    Cost future programmes so that realistic comparisons are made between prison-based programmes and those delivered in the community.
15. *Education, Training and Development*
    Provide comprehensive staff training and development programmes to enable staff to contribute effectively.
16. *Research and Development*
    Establish ongoing research and development programmes to improve service-wide knowledge of what works and to enable objective comparisons between different programmes and establishments to be made.

Research and evaluation

The Evaluation of the Prison Drug Treatment and Rehabilitation report contributed to the formulation of the new Prison Service strategy 'Tackling Drugs in Prison' and builds on the knowledge and experienced gained since 1995 when the original Prison Drug strategy 'Drug Misuse in Prisons' was introduced.

The Prison Service policy is to review current practice as part of its ongoing commitment to measure and evaluate the effectiveness of its drug strategy. This commitment is demonstrated in two further research projects which are examined later in this section – Research into the Nature and Effectiveness of Drug Throughcare and The Home Affairs Committee Report: Drugs and Prisons.

The importance of understanding what works and what provides best value for money is essential if the Government's determination to tackle the supply and use of drugs in prisons is to succeed.

An additional £76 million of funding was made available under the Comprehensive Spending Review for the period 1999 to 2002. This comprises £23.5 million to develop the CARAT service, £17 million to provide places on voluntary testing units and £12.5 million to provide more rehabilitation programmes and increase the provision and accessibility of places in therapeutic communities, especially for women. The remaining £23 million was allocated to improving drug training for staff working in prisons and to improving perimeter security and CCTV in visits rooms, in order to prevent drugs entering penal establishments. (*The Government's Crime Reduction Strategy*, published by The Home Office, November 1999.)

THE EFFECTIVENESS OF DRUG THROUGHCARE

A research project commissioned by the Prison Service in March 1998, titled Research into the Nature and Effectiveness of Drug Throughcare, produced an interim report during 1999 in order that any emerging findings could be incorporated into developing drugs policy. At a time of rapid change, the Prison Service headquarters steering group wanted to maximize the value of any up-to-date evidence-based research. The objectives of the project were twofold: first, to find out what happens to prisoners following release; and second, to establish what works and what influences an offender's drug-taking and pattern of offending.

Methodology

The researchers used a variety of methodologies to achieve their outcomes. These included a survey of professionals, holding focus groups and interviewing the personnel involved in delivering the drugs strategy. These personnel comprised prison and probation staff whose approach was considered progressive; drug services involved in delivering throughcare; and research organizations with previous experience of tracking offenders.

The survey of professionals was conducted in order to examine the role of different agencies in throughcare services and to obtain examples of good practice.

The researchers held a number of focus groups with prisoners to explore their views about how accessible to prisoners are the services provided in prisons; what forms of treatment they had received; and how much support they expected to receive following release.

Interim findings

Despite the challenging nature of this study, a number of general issues emerged that impinge directly on the quality of throughcare.

Resources
(a) A lack of resources is a limiting factor in delivering an effective service as it affects how many suitably trained prison and probation staff are available to deal with drug problems.
(b) Redeploying suitably trained prison officers to cover basic duties results in cancelled appointments.
(c) Adult offenders experience a lack of contact with home probation officers throughout their sentence, which is only resumed shortly before release.
(d) Young offenders feel more positive about their contact with the Probation Service as opposed to social services involvement.
(e) The quality of probation aftercare is generally seen as 'a routine administrative exercise'.
(f) Restricted opportunities exist to be admitted to residential or drug rehabilitation programmes on release.

Co-terminosity
(a) Inter-agency cooperation is made difficult when different agencies do not share geographical boundaries. Since April 2000 the Prison Service area boundaries have become coterminous with the Police and Probation Service administrative boundaries.
(b) Drug Action Teams, social services and health authorities appear to have little commitment to prisoners in custody in their area if they do not normally reside there.
(c) Social services do not contact prisoners outside their area even if they intend to return on release.

Access criteria to local services
(a) Some agencies and local authorities disqualify ex-prisoners from receiving drug services, as in Hammersmith and Fulham in London.

Availability of services
(a) There is uneven provision between penal establishments.
(b) There is a significant shortage of community-based drug rehabilitation services throughout the country.
(c) Lengthy waiting lists for the limited community drug services available means some prisoners relapse in the meantime.

Time available during sentence
(a) Short-term prisoners often cannot receive a needs assessment.
(b) Transferring prisoners between establishments disrupts treatment plans.

Prisoner motivation
(a) Some prisoners refuse to acknowledge they have a drug problem or choose not to tackle their drug misuse, and inevitably continue taking drugs on release.
(b) Relapse prevention is important because some prisoners resume drug-taking within a week to three months of discharge.
(c) Some prisoners would like to transfer to a different area on release to avoid temptation and peer group pressure and to make a fresh start.

Specific issues

The researchers identified several factors within the control of local management that can influence the effective delivery of throughcare services.

Institutional commitment
(a) There needs to be a commitment by prison management to tackle drug problems vigorously.
(b) The drug strategy team should include representatives from throughcare, health care, probation, MDT and a community-based drug agency.
(c) Positive staff attitudes are important if prisoners are to be encouraged to seek help.
(d) At Deerbolt, all personal officers are trained to identify and assess the needs of drug users.
(e) At Full Sutton and Norwich, specialist prison officers on each wing offer advice and liaise with drug agencies.

Identifying drug problems
(a) Making an initial needs assessment, immediately following sentence based on pre-sentence reports, increases the opportunity for involvement in intensive drugs programmes.
(b) At Preston and Wymott, sentence planning targets are recorded on the Local Inmate Data System (LIDS) to help maintain continuity of care.

(c) In Kent, a Transfer of Information document is used to enable information obtained about a prisoner's needs, work undertaken and progress achieved, which moves with the prisoner on transfer.

Sentence management
(a) Although sentence management is an important part of throughcare work with drug misusers, it often does not take place.
(b) Some prisoners are either not included in sentence management or their needs are given a low priority.
(c) Often essential medical information is omitted on the grounds of confidentiality.
(d) A lack of specialist knowledge about drug misuse undermines the effectiveness of sentence plans.
(e) Transferring prisoners because of overcrowding, as opposed to therapeutic considerations, is counterproductive.
(f) Prisoners find agreed objectives set are too generalized and reviews do not take place.

Pre-release courses
(a) Pre-release courses that deal with drug issues and advise prisoners about community drug agencies are valued by them.

Throughcare
(a) Effective throughcare depends on establishing good working relationships between the establishment, the Probation Service and community-based drug agencies.
(b) Ongoing communication is necessary once links are established.

Drugs coordinators
(a) The role of drug coordinator is valuable in making external links before discharge.
(b) This role should be performed by a member of prison staff able to give this work sufficient priority.

Seconded probation officers
(a) Delegating the role of drug coordinator to the seconded probation officer works when there is a probation team operating in the establishment.
(b) Some probation officers lack specialist drug knowledge.
(c) Competing priorities and time constraints mean prisoners on statutory supervision are given priority over those with drug problems.

Prison link officers
(a) Lancashire Probation Service appoints prison link officers who visit prisoners being discharged to addresses in Lancashire and provide a link with local drug rehabilitation support groups.

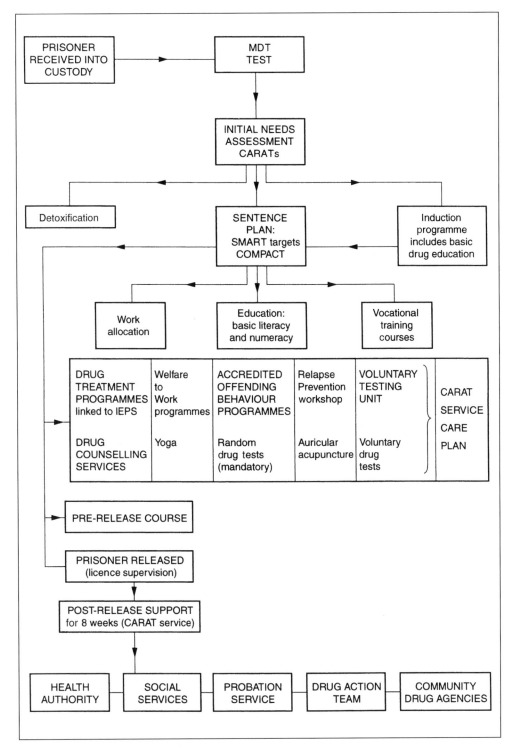

Figure 11: Model of good practice: treatment strategy flowchart

Dedicated drug worker

(a) Coordination works most effectively where a dedicated drug worker is employed directly by the establishment or contracted out to a drug agency.

(b) Drug workers can offer a counselling service, liaise with outside agencies and undertake staff training.

(c) Deerbolt have a dedicated drug worker seconded from the local Probation Service who participates in a community drugs forum.

(d) Prisons in Kent have 'contracts' with Cranstoun and Addaction to follow up 15 per cent of the prisoners they assist in prison, on release.

(e) At Rochester, a dedicated drug worker working with the New Road Project concentrates on a service to remand prisoners, and ensures that anyone who receives a community sentence is seen within 48 hours of their court appearance.

Seamless throughcare

The key to effective throughcare is to define responsibilities clearly between different agencies and nominate dedicated professionals responsible for service delivery. The researchers feel inter-agency cooperation can be improved if efforts are channelled into resolving issues, such as confidentiality vis-à-vis security; becoming involved in joint staff training; developing an 'open door' policy so that prisoners can be seen prior to discharge; and publishing information about the availability of services in each area.

The researchers believed that the new CARAT service has the potential to provide continuity of care and support in the community, in those critical two to three months following release, when relapse is most likely.

Between 1999 and 2002, the Prison Service corporate plan intends to 'establish the effectiveness of the drug strategy through evaluation and research'; this includes evaluating how well the new CARAT services are contributing towards the goal of reducing reoffending.

DRUGS AND PRISONS

The Home Affairs Committee report, Drugs and Prisons, was published on 22 November 1999 and sought to examine the effectiveness of the new prisons drug strategy. The committee conclude their review by stating the strategy is a step in the 'right direction and it provides a platform for progress towards making a period of imprisonment an opportunity for reducing offenders' involvement with drugs'. They highlight six areas of concern that the Prison Service, Home Office and the UK Anti-Drugs Coordinator need to address:

1. Measures should be targeted on the use of hard drugs, as opposed to cannabis.
2. The random mandatory drug testing process needs improving if it is to become a reliable measure of drug use in prisons.
3. Drug detection dogs should be deployed in every prison.

4. The Prison Service should fully utilize the expertise of outside agencies in its treatment programmes.
5. A greater emphasis needs placing on short-term and remand prisoners.
6. The whole drugs strategy could be undermined if there is a shortage of trained drug workers available for prison programmes and the throughcare of prisoners on release.

Conclusions and recommendations

Improvements need to be made to prison regimes
Drug use is more likely to be prevalent in prisons where there is insufficient constructive activity, as prisoners turn to drugs to alleviate boredom. The key performance indicator (KPI) for purposeful activity has fallen from over 26 hours in 1994–5 to under 23 hours in 1998–9. The number of hours prisoners can spend out of their cells has also declined in recent years.

A shortage of qualified drug workers could undermine the strategy
The leading providers of drug treatment services are concerned about the availability of enough trained staff for the new CARAT service. Drug Scope, formerly SCODA, is concerned about the availability of effective treatment services inside and outside prison.

Reducing the supply of drugs is crucial
The overall number of drug finds has fallen from 8561 in 1995, to 5086 in 1998, but more hard drugs are entering prisons because they are less bulky and easier to conceal. In 1998, there were 1079 heroin finds, which has increased from 678 in 1995.

Known drug dealers should be segregated
Insufficient action is being taken to tackle prisoner drug dealers. Greater use could be made of segregation units to curtail their activities, although the Government cautioned against this. The existing system of police liaison officers should be further developed to ensure adequate cover is provided to every establishment. More use could be made of the police advisers section to disseminate intelligence to establishments about know drug dealers who are admitted as visitors or prisoners.

Introduce drug testing of staff where reasonable suspicion exists
Pressure on staff to smuggle drugs and intimidation of their families does occur. Nine staff have been disciplined for drug-related offences in the past six years and three staff resigned after changes were laid.

Random searching of staff
The routine random searching of all staff should take place in every establishment on a more frequent basis.

Improve Visitor Centres
Well-equipped Visitor Centres should be provided where information about drug misuse is freely available. Visitors may be under pressure to supply drugs, and need to be offered support.

Improve CCTV coverage
Extending the use of CCTV in visits areas is known to be effective, but establishments must ensure the monitors are manned at all times by trained staff.

Every establishment should have a passive drug dog
Drug dogs act as an effective deterrent to potential drug smugglers and can detect anyone who has contact with drugs. The numbers deployed are increasing; in April 2000 there were 195 active drug dogs (trained to seek and find substances) and 121 passive drug dogs (who indicate the presence of drugs on visitors and prisoners) – a significant increase. There is scope to use drug dogs more flexibly, such as on random patrols at night, where they can act as a deterrent and as an aid to intelligence-gathering.

Review the standard of searching procedures
There is a pressing need to recruit additional female officers so that all establishments can conduct searches of female visitors to an acceptable standard.

Assess the levels of drug use in prisons
Random MDT results do not accurately reflect the overall level of drug use in an establishment, as the Prison Service has consistently pointed out; it may be considerably higher. Although the available data highlights a downward trend in the use of cannabis, there is no clear downward trend in overall drug use. The level of drug use at 20 per cent is still too high, and there is still disturbing evidence that some prisoners use drugs for the first time whilst in prison. Future research needs to establish whether the MDT programme is reducing the use of cannabis but having no impact on heroin consumption, or even unwittingly encouraging its use.

Differentiate between the use of cannabis and hard drugs
The primary objective of the drugs strategy is to target successfully the use of hard drugs and reduce coincidentally the use of cannabis. Further steps may be necessary to ensure the strategy proves effective in discouraging the use of hard drugs.

Comprehensive Spending Review funding may be insufficient
It is clear that continued funding beyond the present CSR period (1999–2002) will be necessary. The expansion in provision taking place is a major step forward and is reducing the previous inconsistency in delivery across the service.

Treatment programmes need delivering by qualified staff
Treatment programmes should be delivered in partnership with outside providers and coordinated effectively. Prison staff involved in the delivery of treatment programmes

need to receive proper training and become qualified. This means establishing minimum key competencies for staff, and ensuring the training they receive is externally audited. All drug treatment programmes should be accredited and consultations held with outside providers on what the appropriate accreditation criteria should be.

Induction programmes should be more comprehensive
Assessment procedures on reception should be more comprehensive and undertaken by trained staff and health care professionals. Any drug addicts and regular users of hard drugs should be identified on reception, with everybody having to undertake a drug test. There is some inconsistency in the provision of detoxification services and practice relating to prescribing drug substitution medication. However, by early 2002 the number of detoxification units should have increased from 10 to 35. Basic drug education should be part of the induction process for all prisoners, delivered effectively, and the impact continually monitored. More attention needs to be given to remand and short-term prisoners with greater accessibility to drug rehabilitation programmes being provided.

Post-treatment support for prisoners should be provided
Ongoing contact to prisoners, continuing for up to eight weeks after release by the CARAT service providers, is a welcome move in the right direction. It needs supporting by building stronger links between prisoners, the Probation Service and Drug Action Teams. Every prisoner on discharge should have an automatic right of referral to a place on a relevant programme in his home area.

The 'Drug Tsar'

Keith Hellawell, the UK Anti-Drugs Coordinator, is often referred to as the 'Drug Tsar'. He gave evidence to the Home Affairs Committee on 30 March 1999, which is included in the Drugs and Prisons report. He describes his responsibilities to the Committee as to report formally to the Cabinet sub-Committee on Drug Misuse; to produce an Annual Report and Plan; and to coordinate the work of independent Departments and monitor their progress closely. He meets every six to eight weeks with the Home Secretary, the Secretary of State for Health, the Minister responsible for Education and the Foreign Office. He also has direct access to the Prime Minister.

The Home Affairs Committee was concerned to establish the reasons why it appears impossible to stop drugs entering prisons. Keith Hellawell told the committee it would be possible to prevent drugs entering prisons if a totalitarian regime were imposed. This would mean banning open visits with family and friends, as well as subjecting everyone who had any business in the prison to a screening and drug-testing process. However, he believes this would not be an acceptable option in a democratic society.

The availability of drugs
Keith Hellawell told the Committee 'the use of drugs in prison is not as widespread as people might believe', adding that 'the amount of drugs they (prisoners) take is less

than they would normally take outside, because of the limited availability of drugs in prisons'.

Mandatory drug testing

Mandatory drug testing has highlighted the issue of drug misuse in prisons, and helped encourage a positive approach to tackling drugs. Those testing positive for drugs are punished with 'additional penalties on their sentence' (added days), and class A drugs users receive a 'greater additional penalty if they test positive for Class A drugs rather than other drugs'.

Prison treatment programmes

Keith Hellawell views positively the development and growth of drug-free wings (voluntary testing units). He believes introducing drug treatment programmes into prisons will have far-reaching consequences: 'When the strategy begins to bite there will be fewer people going back into prisons because they are not reoffending and going back through the loop.' On the basis of research into the effectiveness of drug treatment programmes in the USA, he maintains that 'For every one pound you put into treatment, the system itself will save about three pounds.'

Improving aftercare arrangements

Keith Hellawell fully recognizes the considerable difficulties in providing effective aftercare for prisoners who successfully complete drug treatment programmes. There is a real danger that prisoners who do not receive the help and support they need on release may quickly relapse and end up back where they started – reoffending to support a drug habit. He sees it as a community problem and identifies prejudice as a major obstacle to delivering effective throughcare: 'There is a strong reluctance in many agencies, many companies, local authorities to provide employment to ex-prisoners anyway. Ex-prisoners who are drug users and drug dealers come right at the bottom of the list.'

Despite the difficulties that face prisoners on release, he welcomes the number of positive initiatives that are taking place in the community: 'New Deal is positive and has a positive impact or influence. We are working with charitable agencies: the Prince's Youth Business Trust, and the Prince's Trust where people want to start their own business.'

Keith Hellawell told the Committee he is currently working with business people throughout the country, charitable agencies and the Drug Action Teams, because 'it is a big problem' and 'we have not got an agency for resettlement'.

The Government's response

The Government's Reply to the Home Affairs Committee report 'Drugs and Prisons' was published on 22nd February 2000. The Government on the whole agrees with the Committee's views, but makes the following points in its reply:

- Supply reduction is a key component of the current drug strategy and a number of steps to reduce the supply of drugs have been taken. These include providing more dogs; extra CCTV; more fixed and low-level furniture.
- The most pressing issue is to create treatment provision across the prison estate. The development of positive regimes in all prisons is a priority task for the Prisons Service.
- The Prison Service intends to fund at least one passive dog in each prison from 2000–01.
- The Government has not seen any evidence which shows that MDT results are unreliable.
- The Government remains committed to preventing the use of all illicit drugs in prisons. It is essential that improvements in the detection and testing of harder drugs does not take place at the expense of detection and testing for cannabis or other drugs considered by some to be less harmful.
- It is crucial that staff involved in providing drug treatment, both prison staff and community drug agency staff, have minimum levels of competence and training. The Prison Service is currently conducting a training-needs analysis to identify an appropriate training framework which ensures all staff working in prisons have appropriate knowledge and skills about drug misuse.
- The case for testing all prisoners on arrival is not straightforward. All drug testing has significant resource implications and there are considerable practical implications for busy local prisons with large numbers of new receptions. Many prisoners coming into custody are aware they have a drug misuse problem, which makes testing everybody a wasteful exercise.
- The Government's view is that prisoners who are serving short sentences are much more likely to be deterred by the prospect of days added to their sentence because of a positive MDT than those serving long sentences. This view contradicts the view expressed by the Committee in paragraph 99 of their report.
- There is no evidence of a shift from cannabis to more harmful drug use in prisons, and the Government rejects the Committee's view expressed in paragraph 108 of the report. While MDT results show a fall in cannabis use, they do not show a rise in the use of other drugs. The MDT programme is only one element in the fight against drug misuse; effective security and good treatment programmes are much more influential.
- The Government agrees that a blanket policy of searching all prisoners in every establishment after visits would not be justified. Such a policy is appropriate for some types of prisoners, and governors have the discretion to impose a blanket policy if they consider on security grounds this is necessary. Searching for drugs is not the only or even the main reason for strip searching prisoners, who must be prevented from bringing into prisons escape equipment, weapons and other prohibited items which could threaten the security or good order of an establishment. Only 2% of prisoners are required to be strip searched after visits and these are category A prisoners and those placed on the escape list. However, there are prisons which either hold high-security prisoners or have a serious drug problem, that consider it appropriate to routinely strip search all prisoners after visits.

- The Government has a long-standing policy that segregation is not used as a punishment. The introduction of the Human Rights Act is likely to endorse this policy. Governors may legitimately segregate prisoners suspected of drug dealing pending an investigation; they may continue that segregation on the authority of a member of the Board of Visitors pending transfer to another establishment.
- The key to eradicating drugs in prisons is a combination of effective security to tackle the supply of drugs, coupled with effective treatment to reduce the demand. The current drug strategy is based on this twin-pronged approach.

DRUG MISUSE RESEARCH

Over 40 per cent of receptions to HMP Bristol admit they have a drug problem. HMP Bristol has developed an effective drugs strategy to combat this problem. It caters for remand and short-term prisoners and provides wing-based detoxification; a voluntary testing unit, comprising 92 beds, offering relapse prevention workshops, yoga, advice and counselling services; and a primary intervention twelve-bedded unit, offering the Primary Intervention Programme (PIP).

The Primary Intervention Programme at HMP Bristol

The Primary Intervention Programme is designed to cater for problem drug users at HMP Bristol. The unit, which is adjacent to the main induction wing, offers a two-week programme which concentrates on increasing the motivation of habitual drug users. The programme has the following aims:

- to increase knowledge and understanding of drug-related issues;
- to explore attitudes and opinions towards drug misuse;
- to equip prisoners with a range of problem-solving and self-management skills.

It covers stress management, problem-solving, setting goals, decision-making and crisis management. In addition, regular auricular acupuncture sessions are used in conjunction with detoxification to encourage quiet reflection.

The programme helps prisoners develop their overall coping skills and ability to handle external pressures, such as negative life events and peer group pressure, and internal pressures, such as anger, anxiety and depression. All those on the unit have urine tests every two days and anyone testing positive loses privileges or is removed from the unit.

An examination of the available data reveals that:

- 43 per cent of applicants were accepted onto the unit, their average age was 29 years, 70 per cent were on remand, and 22 per cent were sentenced prisoners;
- 85 per cent successfully completed the programme; the main reason for failing (8 per cent) was taking drugs on the unit;
- 32 per cent increased their knowledge; test results on the readiness-to-change

questionnaire show that applicants progressed from the contemplation stage, with a score of 4.95 (maximum 8.0), to the action stage, with a score of 6.29, on completion of the programme.

These results demonstrate the programme has achieved some success in meeting the stated aims. Although many prisoners are managing to avoid a relapse whilst in prison and immediately after release, the lack of good quality aftercare means a significant number are drifting back into a criminal drug culture.

IDENTIFYING BEST PRACTICE

The Prison Service has developed a comprehensive set of standards for service delivery which includes the implementation of the drugs strategy. Overall performance is monitored by the Standards Audit Team who visit each establishment biannually and report their findings to the Governor and headquarters. They assess the drug strategy module against a set of baselines. The overall level of compliance is presently classified in one of five categories: Superior, Good, Acceptable, Deficient, Unacceptable.

Auditing the drugs strategy

The module on the drugs strategy requires compliance by an establishment with a comprehensive set of baselines. In order to meet the auditor's requirements it is necessary for staff to produce supporting documentation and answer the following questions about drugs practice in the establishment:

1. Has a comprehensive local drugs strategy been devised by the Governor and agreed with the Area Manager?
2. Is responsibility for implementing the strategy allocated to a multi-disciplinary team led by a senior manager?
3. Does the drugs strategy coordinator lead the multi-disciplinary drug strategy team and are a wide range of departments, external agencies and the CARAT service provider represented?
4. Have the drugs strategy team made a comprehensive assessment of local needs together with an evaluation of the resources available to deal with drug misuse?
5. Are systems in place to prevent drugs being smuggled into the prison including the searching of prisoners and visitors?
6. What measures have been introduced to deal effectively with prisoners believed to be involved in drug smuggling through visits?
7. Are passive drugs dogs being used in the visits area?
8. Has the establishment installed CCTV and low-level furniture in the visits room?
9. Is there a system for booking visits in advance?
10. Does the local drugs strategy have a detailed implementation plan, which incorporates target dates and regular reviews?

11. Has the establishment developed partnerships with relevant community-based agencies?
12. Does the drug-testing programme ensure an agreed proportion of the population are tested each month?
13. Has a voluntary testing unit been established which contains a discrete testing suite?
14. Have all the sample takers attended the appropriate training course?
15. Do staff issue the MDT authorization form to all prisoners before conducting a test?
16. Is the correct chain of custody followed when conducting random tests, targeted mandatory tests and voluntary tests?
17. Does the MDT coordinator use the LIDS Random Number Generation System each month to identify prisoners for random testing?
18. Is there a system in place for identifying and authorizing 'on suspicion' tests, risk assessments and those on the frequent testing programme?
19. Are all prisoners who refuse to provide a urine sample charged with a disciplinary offence?
20. Is every prisoner who tests positive offered suitable advice and guidance?
21. Has a suitable system been introduced that identifies those prisoners with a drug problem and ensures that a needs assessment and CARAT care plan is prepared?
22. Are a range of suitable treatment programmes available?
23. Is harm reduction information available?
24. Are drug awareness classes provided for prisoners?
25. Does the local staff training programme include sessions on drug education?

The Standards Audit Unit findings

The Standards Audit Annual Report 1996–1999 concluded that the service has much to be proud of in this area. The most recent audit year coincided with the implementation of the Prison Service drugs strategy, 'Tackling Drugs in Prison'.

The Standards Audit Team found 90.6 per cent of establishments audited achieved a rating of Acceptable or better and 59.4 per cent of establishments warranted a Good or better rating.

Two main shortcomings need to be addressed: the operation of multi-disciplinary drug strategy teams in establishments; and the lack of timed implementation plans to support the local drugs strategy.

Good practice

The audit report highlights good practice in many establishments in respect of:

- procedures to prevent drugs entering establishments;
- the quality of mandatory drug testing;
- the range of drug treatment programmes available;
- the availability of information, advice, guidance and drug education;

- involvement in multi-agency partnerships within the local community;
- good local staff training.

In 1999, the following establishments received a 'Superior' rating by the Standards Audit Team because there was impressive evidence of best practice in delivering the drugs strategy: Belmarsh; Elmley; Liverpool; Long Lartin; Lowdham Grange; North-allerton; and Swinfen Hall.

COST-EFFECTIVENESS OF TREATMENT PROGRAMMES

Research conducted in the USA indicates that drug treatment programmes are cost-effective. In California, the Department of Alcohol and Drug Programmes studied how beneficial drug treatment programmes were to the 1850 persons who had participated. They published their findings in 1994. Their conclusion that providing drug treatment programmes is cost-effective is based on the following findings:

- *Crime reduction*
  The crime-rate reduced by two-thirds when making comparisons about the level of offending before and after treatment.
- *Health improved*
  Significant improvements in the health of those participating occurred.
- *Hospital admissions reduced*
  There were reductions in the numbers requiring hospital in-patient care.
- *Criminal activity reduced*
  The incidence of offending reduced sharply whilst individuals were under-going treatment, which demonstrates that treatment programmes are self-financing.

The researchers argue that every £1 spent providing drug treatment programmes gives a return on the investment worth £7. The financial cost of placing 150,000 persons in drug treatment programmes in the state of California was $209 million. The cost benefits that arose during the time they spent undergoing treatment and in the following year amounted to savings for the taxpayer of $1.5 billion.

Prison Service programmes

The Prison Service is assessing the potential cost-effectiveness of offending behaviour programmes which are currently being financed by CSR funding for the period 1999 to 2002.

Research conducted in Canada and the USA has identified the key factors that are fundamental to undertaking effective work with offenders, and they are as follows:

- programmes that concentrate on addressing
  - (a) anti-social behaviour,
  - (b) drug dependency,
  - (c) limited cognitive skills,
  - (d) poor interpersonal skills,
  - (e) improving educational and vocational basic skills;
- using well trained staff to deliver programmes;
- delivering structured programmes using an active, participative approach;
- developing the problem-solving abilities of prisoners;
- targeting intensive programmes at high-risk offenders.

Providing that these conditions are met, the cost-effectiveness of programmes can result in a 10 per cent reduction in reconvictions.

The data that follows is based on a number of assumptions derived from the experience of those running programmes in Canada and the USA. In Great Britain there is little evidence based on programmes run by the Prison Service due to the 'nothing works' culture prevalent in the 1980s.

The Crime Reduction Strategy

The Government's Crime Reduction Strategy, published in November 1999, explains why it is investing an additional £76 million to tackle drug misuse, and outlines how it intends to spend this additional funding:

- an increase in assessment and treatment services for drug users;
- more units for prisoners wishing to avoid taking drugs;
- an increase in drug training for staff working in prisons;
- improved security to prevent drugs entering establishments.

The report estimates that drug testing, assessment and referral services could reduce recorded crime by around 25,000 incidences in 2001–2.

The Prison Service drugs strategy aims to treat the majority of prisoners who have a drug problem. Approximately 120,000 prisoners come into custody each year, half of whom have a drug problem. Around 4000 (6 per cent) have a serious crime-related drug problem and the Prison Service expects to achieve a 25 per cent reduction in reconviction rates for this group. They calculate the following reductions in reconviction rates can be achieved:

- Accredited Offending Behaviour programmes   10 per cent
- Improving Basic Literacy and Numeracy Skills   10 per cent
- Welfare to Work programmes   10 per cent
- High Intensity Regimes for juveniles   10 per cent

These calculations are based on delivering the following planned programmes during the period 1999–2002:

Table 2: Reducing reconviction rates

	Total throughput 1999–2002	Assumed reduction in reconvictions	Numbers expected to be prevented from offending	Expected number of offences prevented based on 5 recorded offences per person*
Accredited programmes (excluding Sex Offender Treatment Programmes)	14,400	10%	1,440	7,200
Drugs strategy	180,000	25%	3,000	75,000
Basic literacy and numeracy (estimate of additional numbers achieving Level 2)	15,750	10%	1,575	7,875
Welfare to Work	7,500	10%	750	3,750
Juvenile regimes	15,000	5%	750	3,750

*Except for the drugs strategy, where the assumption is 25 offences per person

The Drugs Strategy 1999–2002

The Prison Service calculates that the drugs strategy will prevent 3000 prisoners committing 75,000 offences. The cost of each recorded offence is £1333, and this brings a saving for each offence of £1157 as a benefit to society. This figure is arrived at from conducting a number of complex mathematical calculations adjusted to take into account the pattern of offending on discharge and sentences handed out by the courts on first reconviction to discharged prisoners. Based on these assumptions, the Prison Service drugs strategy alone for 1999–2002 could bring savings to society of 75,000 offences saved × £1157 benefit per offence = £86.7 million, equivalent to £28.9 million per annum.

CHECKLIST

- What are the three main proven benefits of providing treatment and rehabilitation programmes?
- Why is the RAPt twelve-steps programme at HMP Downview particularly effective?
- How do you evaluate the success of a drug treatment programme?
- What is the link between crime and drug misuse?
- Are residential programmes effective in treating heroin users?
- How effective are methadone maintenance and methadone reduction programmes?
- Why is drug misuse described as a 'chronic relapsing condition'?
- What problems face those wanting to access community drug services?
- How does the lack of co-terminosity make inter-agency cooperation more difficult?
- What is seamless throughcare?
- How can the Prison Service further improve its drug treatment and rehabilitation services?
- Which two groups of prisoners have most difficulty receiving help with a drug problem?
- What action can Governors take to tackle known drug dealers?
- When should drug testing of prison staff be carried out?
- How can a passive drug dog be used as an aid to intelligence-gathering?
- Does improving prison regimes help counter drugs use?
- Why are more hard drugs entering prisons?
- Is the MDT programme reducing heroin use in prisons?
- Why should all discharged prisoners have an 'automatic right of referral' to a place on a relevant programme in their home areas?
- Would a totalitarian regime in prisons prevent drugs entering prisons?
- Is a totalitarian approach politically acceptable?
- Why does the UK Anti-Drugs Coordinator believe the Prison Service drugs strategy will result in 'fewer people going back into prisons'?
- Prejudice is a major obstacle to delivering effective throughcare. Who are the main culprits?
- How does the Standards Audit Unit assess the effectiveness of the drugs strategy?
- What research evidence supports the view that drug treatment programmes are cost-effective?
- Why does the Prison Service believe the drugs strategy can prevent 3000 prisoners committing 75,000 offences?

CHAPTER 9

Reviewing Performance

HER MAJESTY'S CHIEF INSPECTOR OF PRISONS

Assessing the effectiveness of a new policy takes time. An objective way to determine the impact of 'Tackling Drugs in Prison' is to examine a representative sample of HMCIP reports of inspections conducted during 1999 and published the same year. They provide an up-to-date picture of how consistently the drug strategy is being implemented in establishments across the country, although it must be borne in mind that the CARAT service did not commence until 1 October 1999.

The following inspections and reports are arranged in chronological order as follows:

Prison	Inspection	Report published
HMP Liverpool	18–27 January	17 June
HMP Wymott	22–26 February	22 July
HMP Wormwood Scrubs	8–12 March	13 July
HMYOI Huntercombe	23–25 March	16 June
HMP Highdown	2–4 and 30 March	13 July
HMP Bristol	12–21 April	20 July
HMYOI and RC Reading	19–23 April	5 October
HMP and YOI Parc	10–19 May	14 October
HMP Exeter	17–26 May	12 August
HMP and YOI Bullwood Hall	24–27 May	27 October
HMP Preston	14–23 June	15 October
HMYOI Hatfield	19–23 June	2 December
HMP Wayland	2–3 August	2 November
HMP and HMYOI Hollesley Bay Colony	23–25 August	8 December

HMP LIVERPOOL

Liverpool is the largest prison in England and Wales with a population of 1500. Although described as a local prison – it only has 300 prisoners on remand and a population of 1200 sentenced prisoners – it operates like a large training prison. The main offence of 17.6 per cent of the prisoners is drug-related.

What prisoners said

A group of unsentenced prisoners told the inspectors:

- all prisoners are treated with suspicion, as though they were drug addicts;
- they want a drug-free wing so they can distance themselves from the drug culture.

A group of sentenced prisoners told the inspectors:

- prisoners strongly resent having to share cells with class A drug abusers;
- there is a six-month waiting list for the drugs course;
- they feel the drugs course patronizes them;
- the tutors know less about drugs than the prisoners do.

What the Governor said

The Governor said no funding was made available for the local drug strategy until October 1997 when two health care workers were appointed. The Board of Visitors endorsed the view that there is a drugs problem with too few resources available to tackle it.

The drugs strategy

The inspectors felt the scale of the drug problem facing Liverpool is intransigent. The majority of prisoners have a history of abusing class A drugs (heroin and cocaine) and nearly 80 per cent of them have a history of drug-taking.

Although MDT was operating satisfactorily, opportunities for treatment are very restricted. Since the drugs strategy has been introduced, the establishment have introduced a drug clinic, a drug throughcare team and employed a drug liaison officer.

Reception
On reception prisoners are given information about the range of services available in the prison. Many prisoners decline to disclose they have a drug problem in case they are targeted for MDT testing.

The inspectors recommend prisoners are able to access drug services throughout their sentence, and those wishing to admit officially that they are drug users are able to receive confidential advice and support.

Health care
Prisoners with a drug problem are referred to the drug clinic based in the health care centre. The inspectors found the dispensing arrangements are being abused and the medical officer has no experience or training in working with drug abusers. Offering

hepatitis B vaccinations to prisoners is being discouraged owing to budgetary pressure.

The inspectors feel the size of the drug problem merits additional staffing and funding to develop a comprehensive health care service.

Throughcare

The appointment of a drug liaison officer enables good community links to become established and referral systems to rehabilitation programmes in other prisons to take place.

The probation and education departments provide groupwork services; prison officers are involved in delivering drug-related groups and the RC Chaplain runs a religious twelve-steps programme.

The drug throughcare team is managed by Arch Initiatives (an external voluntary group) who concentrate on the needs of remand prisoners and sentenced prisoners serving up to twelve months. They deliver training to wing-based prison officers and provide a number of groups. Arch Initiatives have considerable expertise in assessment and referral services and perform an invaluable aftercare role by helping ex-prisoners access community-based drug services.

MDT

MDT is conducted efficiently in a discrete and dedicated MDT suite in a way that does not reduce a prisoner's dignity. The percentage of positive random tests conducted in the previous year (1998) was 23 per cent.

The number of 'on suspicion' tests was considerably higher. This indicates that reducing the availability of drugs needs tackling more vigorously and the level of targeted drug tests need increasing.

A serious weakness in the system is an absence of drug testing at weekends.

Voluntary testing units

HMP Liverpool does not have a voluntary testing unit or arrangements in place for conducting voluntary tests. It is recommended that a VTU is set up with support on relapse prevention built into the regime.

Overall findings

The inspectors found many aspects of the drug strategy positive. Their concerns centre on the lack of coordination, the competing nature of services, and the absence of any quality control systems or mechanisms in place to evaluate the effectiveness of services being provided.

They recommend that the drug strategy group takes responsibility for coordinating the strategy and ensuring it is evidence-based. The role of the drug strategy group is to agree, develop and manage the available resources effectively. They need to be more directive and to review actively all drug-related issues.

The level of existing resources is described as 'woefully inadequate', with major areas of unmet need likely to remain despite the injection of CSR funding.

They recommend the Area Drug Coordinator assesses the level of resources necessary to meet the standards contained in the Prison Service strategy and advises Prison Service Headquarters accordingly.

HMP WYMOTT

HMP Wymott has an operational capacity of 805. It operates as two separate establishments within the same perimeter, with two distinct staff groups running different regimes under a single management.

The main prison is a modern category C training prison comprising 365 prisoners. The Vulnerable Prisoner Unit (VPU) comprises 440 sex offenders who are housed in older inferior accommodation. The main offence of 22.5 per cent of the prisoners is drug-related.

What prisoners said

A group of vulnerable prisoners told the inspectors:

- they do not receive an induction programme;
- they are locked away and forgotten about;
- staff attitudes are hostile;
- sentence management boards are intimidating.

A group of category C prisoners told the inspectors:

- visitors experience lengthy delays before visits commence;
- too many visitors receive a strip search based on indications by the passive drug dog.

The drugs strategy

HMP Wymott has a significant drug misuse problem amongst the category C population with 50 to 70 per cent having a history of serious drug abuse. Amongst the VPU prisoners, drug misuse is minimal and restricted to a few individuals.

There is little evidence that a needs analysis has been conducted. The drugs strategy document needs revising and updating and making relevant to those involved in delivering the strategy locally. A drug practitioners group is operating and gives support to staff working directly with prisoners.

Reception

All prisoners are screened by a health care worker and seen by the medical officer or duty doctor within 24 hours.

Health care
Health care is not represented on the drugs strategy team or involved in delivering services to prisoners with drug-related infectious diseases. The fifteen prisoners who are hepatitis C positive are believed to be the tip of the iceberg.

The inspectors feel testing and treatment options for prisoners need expanding and developing as a matter of urgency. More programmes should be targeted on harm reduction and addressing drug education needs.

Throughcare
A specialist part-time drugs worker, contracted in from 'Lifeline', is involved in staff training. Lifeline provide an induction group, and an assessment, advice and referral service.

The probation team run a six-week drug-related Offending Behaviour programme of 24 sessions, similar in content to accredited offending behaviour programmes. They deliver five to six programmes a year, catering up to ten prisoners on each course.

MDT
The percentage of positive random tests conducted in the previous year (1998) in the category C units was 31.1 per cent compared to 3.3 per cent in the VPU. The number of heroin positive results among the category C population is well above average, supporting the belief that large numbers of prisoners have serious drug problems.

Voluntary testing units
Prisoners with no previous history of drug use and no inclination to take drugs, need protecting from the prevailing drug culture. It is apparent a VTU is desperately needed supported by a CARAT scheme.

The inspectors found staff keen to become involved in delivering the drugs strategy with some already working in partnership with other specialists.

Overall findings

The inspectors recommend the drug strategy team is chaired by a more senior manager and the published strategy revised and updated.

The number of drug-related Offending Behaviour programmes needs expanding and the content of drug programmes widened to include drug education and prevention, and harm reduction.

The inspectors are convinced that the level of resources available to tackle drugs effectively is inadequate, although CSR funding should make a difference.

The Area Manager should base his decisions about resource allocation on the principle of ensuring prisoners in the north-west area have equal access to drug services.

HMP WORMWOOD SCRUBS

Wormwood Scrubs is the best known prison in the UK and accommodates 890 prisoners on five wings. A wing has unsentenced prisoners; B wing sentenced prisoners, the segregation unit and the Vulnerable Prisoner Unit; C wing is closed for refurbishment; D wing contains sentenced prisoners; and E wing lifers.

At the time of the inspection, the Crown Prosecution Service were investigating several allegations of ill treatment made by prisoners against staff.

What prisoners said

A group of unsentenced prisoners told the inspectors:

*   A wing is chaotic with no set routine;
*   association is restricted to the ground floor which reduces the risk of bullying;
*   health care screening by the medical officer is cursory.

A group of sentenced prisoners told the inspectors:

*   there is no personal officer scheme;
*   one officer is brutal and rips up applications;
*   the results of the MDT are not trusted;
*   whilst drugs are not readily available, there is more cannabis than heroin in circulation.

A group of lifers on E wing told the inspectors:

*   courses on Anger Management and Enhanced Thinking Skills are often cancelled;
*   staff are lazy, demoralized and apathetic.

The drugs strategy

HMP Wormwood Scrubs has not analysed the scale of the drugs misuse problem, although what evidence is available points to there being a significant problem. An assessment in 1998 by the detoxification unit identified 655 prisoners with a drug problem, of whom 132 (20 per cent) were admitted to the unit. The true figure is probably higher because many prisoners are reluctant to admit to having a drug problem.

The drug strategy committee, chaired by a governor grade, is active and includes representatives from all the relevant agencies and staff dealing with drug misuse in the prison.

Reception

New receptions are not advised about the prison routines and the induction programme is virtually non-existent. Nor are they seen by the medical officer until 1700 hours that day.

Health care

The health care service acts as a national resource to treat very sick and disturbed prisoners. Ward H3 can cater for 30 patients with mental health problems and has a eight-bed detoxification unit comprising a four-bed dormitory and four single cells, one of which has been unusable for over a year due to maintenance problems.

The inspectors found the detoxification unit in need of redecoration and general refurbishment. It does not have a kitchen and food is stored in an office.

There is no clear criteria for making referrals to the detoxification unit and most decisions to admit are taken by health care staff on reception without any apparent consultation. In a six-month period, 88 prisoners were admitted for drug detoxification, 20 for alcohol addictions and 6 for dual addictions.

Staff on the detoxification unit face the following difficulties:

- limited staff available to run a substance misuse link-nurse pilot project which supports prisoners on residential wings;
- the unit is inadequately staffed;
- exercise is frequently cancelled because staffing levels on the unit have been reduced;
- the detoxification unit is failing to deliver the regime outlined in the prisoner compact.

Throughcare

Drug services in the prison are provided by four voluntary agencies. They provide assessment, referral and throughcare services for two days a week. This service is not coordinated and lacks consistency, prompting the inspectors to suggest involving fewer agencies might be beneficial.

Hammersmith and Fulham community health team provide a quality targeted service to prisoners, addressing HIV/AIDS and drug problems.

Problems associated with hepatitis infection are not tackled effectively and the drug strategy team are urged to examine how appropriate testing, treatment and support services can be provided.

The prison-based probation team provide the link between specialist voluntary workers and the home probation officer. They provide a service to the detoxification unit and residential wings.

MDT

Positive random tests make up 28.8%, of which 18.5% are positive results for cannabis and 6.9% for opiates. The other 3.4% are made up by other illegal substances tested for in the laboratory.

Prison officers have little involvement in the drug strategy and the inadequacy of resources seriously undermines the ability of staff to tackle drug misuse problems effectively:

- staff have not been trained to operate CCTV in the visits area;
- staff are redeployed from searching to other duties;

- cell searching targets are not met;
- only 53 drug finds were made over a six-month period;
- class A users frequently escape detection because of delays in carrying out 'on suspicion' MDT tests.

Voluntary testing units

Adjacent to the hospital is the Max Glatt Centre, a 32-bed therapeutic community which treats addictive behaviour. Nearly all of the residents have drug misuse problems. Therapeutic groups are run by specialist therapists, with full community meetings taking place twice a week. One therapy group uses a range of cognitive-behavioural interventions like relapse prevention and anger management for substance abusers. Accredited Social and Life Skill classes are provided, but the Enhanced Thinking course and quarterly case conferences have ceased. Despite the lack of psychological input for over two years, the unit is valued by prisoners who value the help they receive with their problems.

The Max Glatt Centre has developed a therapeutic culture: staff have a positive attitude to treatment; they are highly committed and they have counselling skills.

Overall findings

The inspectors recommend the drugs strategy committee carry out a comprehensive needs analysis and develop an effective strategy, which should be published and used to evaluate overall performance and the programmes provided.

The security department is not addressing the problem of drugs entering the establishment effectively.

The detoxification unit must be staffed appropriately to provide the agreed regime.

Prison staff must be trained and actively involved in delivering the drugs strategy.

HMYOI HUNTERCOMBE

Huntercombe is a Young Offender Institution which comprises five houseblocks and has a Certified Normal Accommodation (CNA) of 360.

The main offence of 8.9 per cent of the young offenders and juveniles is drug-related.

What prisoners said

A group of juveniles told the inspectors:

- there is no real counselling offered to those with drug and alcohol problems;
- it is hard to get a place on the Drug and Alcohol Awareness course (it can take up to twelve months);
- drug testing is always 'on suspicion'; no random testing takes place.

A group of young offenders told the inspectors:

* offending behaviour courses are available;
* offending behaviour courses are oversubscribed and waiting lists are long;
* the prison-based and outside probation officers do not talk to each other.

What the Governor said

His vision is to provide a structure of care for individuals in the establishment by breaking the population down into smaller groups. He interviews each new reception and sees them on discharge to assess what has been achieved with them whilst in custody. These interviews are written up, and the inspectors commend this as an outstanding example of good practice.

The Board of Visitors said staff recruitment and retention is a major problem.

The drugs strategy

The inspectors make no reference to the drugs strategy since the focus of the short inspection was to examine progress on recommendations from the last inspection carried out in May 1994.

The procedure for dealing with applications for Release on Temporary Licence (ROTL) was examined. At the ROTL board, the young offenders are warned about the pressure they may come under from other inmates to bring drugs back into the establishment.

Reception
The reception area has been redesigned, but it remains austere and contains a small medical interview room which does not safeguard prisoner confidentiality.

Health care
Many of the youngsters have complex psychological and emotional problems and are offered counselling. There is a huge demand for this service but the counsellor is only employed on one day a week.

A pilot study has revealed that many of the juveniles have an Attention Deficit Disorder (ADD) or a Attention Deficit Hyperactivity Disorder (ADHD). It is planned to address this need through a programme run by a psychologist and a psychiatrist, and by using health care staff.

Throughcare
Anger management, victim awareness and drug and alcohol courses are provided by the probation team. The Drug Awareness course is appreciated but is criticized for not being sufficiently comprehensive. This course is not being evaluated and there is concern about the excessive waiting lists that exist which indicate the need for additional resources.

Prison officers and probation officers jointly deliver a Crime and Consequences course in the drama studio, and the senior psychologist is setting up an Enhanced Thinking Skills for prison staff to run. However, none of the courses provided are accredited.

A shared drug worker provides an individual counselling service and makes referrals for aftercare services prior to their release.

MDT
No information is available on random testing.

Voluntary testing units
There are no voluntary testing or drug-free facilities.

Overall findings

Huntercombe has limited counselling facilities and no therapeutic programmes for youngsters with drug or alcohol dependency problems. Programmes need introducing that provide help for young people with substance abuse problems.

The Offending Behaviour courses provided should be evaluated and adequate resources provided to cater for identified need.

Family meetings are arranged to identify and deal with any discharge needs; this is good practice. Close liaison is maintained with youth justice workers.

HMP HIGHDOWN

HMP Highdown opened in 1992 at a cost of £91 million. It is a local prison that contains up to 40 category A prisoners. It has a Certified Normal Accommodation of 649 but at the time of the inspectors' visits contained 751 prisoners including fourteen lifers.

Thirty-one per cent of the population are on remand or unsentenced, and the main offence of 20.3 per cent of the prisoners is drug-related.

The drugs strategy

The inspectors make no reference to the drugs strategy as they focused on progress made in implementing the recommendations from the inspection conducted in April 1995, which predates the new drugs strategy 'Tackling Drugs in Prison'.

Reception
Procedures for screening new receptions are very poor, with prisoners frequently moved from reception without seeing a health care worker. This practice is potentially dangerous as it places unscreened prisoners at risk.

Health care
There are serious shortcomings with existing health care arrangements due to staffing shortfalls and management problems. As a result, no need assessments for health care services are carried out, nor are prisoners with drug misuse problems identified.

Throughcare
A multi-disciplinary throughcare policy group meet quarterly under the chairmanship of the Deputy Governor. Offending behaviour courses are run by probation officers who review and evaluate them using feedback forms. It is planned to run accredited courses funded from CSR money.

MDT
No information is available on random testing.

Voluntary testing units
A voluntary drugs testing unit is based in one of the houseblocks formerly used as a resettlement unit. Although its capacity is limited, it is an encouraging start and offers prisoners a 'substance-free' environment.

Overall findings

The effect of serious staffing shortfalls means some basic tasks are not being carried out; this neutralizes the value of CSR funding.

A systematic needs analysis of all prisoners should be carried out and offending behaviour courses provided to address identified need.

The induction programme needs to be reviewed and the personal officer scheme extended to all prisoners.

HMP BRISTOL

HMP Bristol is a Victorian local prison with a population of 580. The prisoners are accommodated in five wings, one of which acts as an induction unit and detoxification unit. Remand prisoners make up 34 per cent of the population; a further 19.5 per cent are convicted but not sentenced. The main offence of 7.5 per cent of the prisoners is drug-related.

What prisoners said

A group of remand and unconvicted prisoners told the inspectors:

- staff on visits are over-suspicious and paranoid;
- staff are slow to answer cell bells.

A group of lifers told the inspectors that prisoners testing positive for MDT are placed on closed visits for three months and must have a clear MDT before normal visits can resume.

A group of Category A prisoners told the inspectors that babies and visitors are regularly searched.

The drugs strategy

HMP Bristol is developing an impressive drugs strategy. A comprehensive needs analysis is carried out on all new receptions, with effective detoxification strategies in place to tackle those with drug problems.

The medical officer identified 1016 new receptions using heroin, of which 64 per cent were injecting, and including 411 prisoners who were using crack/cocaine. High numbers of prisoners use benzodiazepines and amphetamines, whilst polydrug use is widespread. A further study identified 548 out of 1289 new receptions (42.5 per cent) with a drug problem. Ninety per cent of them (495) admitted they used heroin immediately prior to imprisonment.

The drugs strategy team meet bimonthly and comprise the senior management group. The team are developing good links with the local community, and representatives attend the Drug Action Team and Drug Reference Group. The establishment have considerable expertise in detoxification and combating drugs, and the existing treatment programmes are commended as examples of good practice.

Reception

A comprehensive induction programme is provided which lasts two days. It could be further improved by the inclusion of a session of harm reduction in relation to drugs and alcohol abuse.

Sentence plans are carried out to an exceptionally high standard with annual reviews and documentation completed on time by a dedicated group of staff.

Prisoners are encouraged to address their drug problems and are seen by the medical officer and a nurse on reception, who assess all drug users and refer them for treatment. A leaflet, Drugs and You, is given to all new receptions which explains what help is available in prison. HMP Bristol offers harm-reduction programmes, support services on release and a detoxification programme.

The detoxification programme is 'extremely advanced and sophisticated' and in the previous year, 18 per cent of the population received a medical detox. Post-detoxification support is available from nursing staff.

Health care

The Primary Intervention Unit offer a three-week programme catering for ten prisoners who wish to adopt a drug-free lifestyle. The programme adopts a cognitive-behavioural approach to motivate prisoners and works closely with outside agencies. Prisoners value the programme finding it challenging and stimulating.

A peer support training programme is offered to prisoners having the skills and motivation to help other prisoners.

Health awareness promotion about hepatitis is proving effective. A recent study revealed that 24 per cent of the prisoners having blood tests had tested positive for hepatitis C.

Throughcare
A multi-disciplinary approach to throughcare is taken and a range of offending behaviour programmes are available to prisoners. The psychology department is developing programmes with the probation team and taking the lead in delivering cognitive skills programmes. The probation team offer programmes to prisoners on remand and those serving short sentences.

Several drug agencies run groups including the Southmead and Bristol Drugs Project and the Bridge House Hostel. The establishment intends to have sixteen courses operational during 2000. At the time of the inspection they were providing: acupuncture, yoga, employment advice, drug awareness, individual counselling sessions, handling emotions, a group for crack cocaine users and a course provided by the Southmead and Bristol Drug Project.

Close links have been formed with other parts of the criminal justice system in the Bristol area, including drug workers in other agencies.

MDT
MDT is carried out efficiently by a team of trained officers and the target of 10 per cent random tests is consistently achieved. The percentage of positive random tests conducted in the previous year (1998) was 25 per cent with cannabis the most commonly detected drug found in 15 per cent of all random samples.

The first three months of 1999 show a significant reduction in the level of positive random tests, to under 12 per cent. This coincides with the introduction of improved security measures targeted at visitors which are proving very effective: 40 visitors were detected attempting to bring drugs into the establishment.

Voluntary testing units
C wing is designated a drug-free wing and contains 60–70 convicted short-term prisoners, two-thirds of whom have a history of drug misuse. Any prisoner seeking help to tackle his drug problem is admitted to the unit providing he signs a compact agreeing to have regular drug tests. However, little voluntary drug testing is taking place and the inspectors recommend regular voluntary drug testing is introduced to enhance the credibility of the VTU.

Each prisoner is given an information sheet outlining the range of services available to help him tackle drug misuse problems. These include: individual counselling sessions, discussion groups and gaining practical skills.

Two prison officers act as drug support workers, interviewing and assessing all applicants for suitability for the VTU. The inspectors feel, with appropriate training, their role could be widened to include providing casework and groupwork support to prisoners.

Overall findings

The inspectors found several examples of good practice during their inspection:

- they highlight the extent to which HMP Bristol is in advance of many prisons with its drug strategy;
- the staff providing throughcare services are commended for their vision and drive;
- the detoxification programme is extremely advanced and sophisticated;
- excellent work is being done to promote awareness about hepatitis.

The inspectors made several recommendations including:

- the budget for detoxification should be reviewed;
- prisoners undergoing detox should not be separated from the rest of the population but offered a programme which motivates and supports them;
- coordination and collaboration between those providing treatment programmes and health care services could be improved;
- more suitable accommodation should be provided for drug-based programmes within the prison.

HMYOI AND RC READING

Reading is a remand centre for young offenders with a CNA of 203 and an operational capacity of 245. Thirty-six per cent of the population are unsentenced and 11 per cent are juveniles, aged 17. The main offence of 4.37 per cent of the youngsters at Reading is drug-related.

What prisoners said

A group of convicted youngsters told the inspectors:

- anyone caught trying to smuggle drugs is placed on closed visits;
- the time spent on closed visits is not specified;
- strip searches are not carried out on a random basis; anyone with a 'dodgy face' is targeted.

A group of remand youngsters told the inspectors that there are very few drugs in the prison and that drug addicts are given anti-depressants for about a month.

A group of juveniles told the inspectors:

- it is a safe establishment;
- visitors who try to smuggle drugs are targeted;
- prisoners caught trafficking get 21 days added to their sentence.

What the Governor said

The Governor's vision is to have a well-ordered regime within a clean environment. He believes CSR funding can enhance the regime by providing resources for an Enhanced Thinking Skills accredited course. Good external links exist with several agencies involved with drug misusers.

The Board of Visitors are concerned about the level of drugs in the establishment, but praises the work of ACORN, a local drugs agency working in Reading.

The drugs strategy

The drugs strategy committee meet quarterly and have a policy document which focuses on reducing supply, on drug detection and on offering counselling services. A needs analysis should be conducted to assess the scale of drug misuse at Reading.

A recent bid for a detoxification and rehabilitation unit has been approved to help remand prisoners with drug dependency problems.

The establishment has two staff trainers in drug awareness but new staff are not receiving drug awareness training.

There is an over-reliance on CCTV in the visits room and as a result visitors are not being searched. Amnesty bins are being provided to discourage visitors from bringing drugs into visits.

A drug dog is no longer used, but a bid for CSR funding for a passive and active drug dog has been approved.

Reception
ACORN provide a drugs counsellor to interview all new receptions and are to be given a 'slot' in the induction programme. This encourages closer links with health care services and provides an opportunity to give young offenders information about hepatitis C and HIV. A good practice that has been introduced is a 'drop-in' centre, held once a week in the association room, which allows youngsters access to help and advice. A rolling programme of groupwork is provided for those who want to tackle their problems. It already has a four-week waiting list.

Health care
Initial health care screening is carried out on reception by nursing staff, and the medical officer sees them the following day. Receptions can arrive any time up to 20:00 hours, so additional medical support is being contracted in to enable a medical assessment to take place on arrival.

The inspectors consider that needs assessments should be introduced as a priority.

Throughcare
The head of throughcare is a governor grade. He manages the senior probation officer but is not responsible for the sentence planning unit. The inspectors recommend that a psychology unit is established under the leadership of a chartered senior psychologist to deliver accredited offending behaviour programmes. CSR funding has been made

available to recruit a treatment manager to provide an Enhanced Thinking Skills course.

MDT

MDT is conducted in a dedicated suite on a wing which is in a dreadful state. There is building debris and dust everywhere caused by building work which is in progress. These health, hygiene and safety issues need addressing as a matter of urgency because the MDT suite is considered unusable in this state.

Young prisoners who fail an MDT are placed on closed visits for one month. Anyone found in possession of drugs is placed on closed visits for three months. This policy is illogical and needs to be reviewed.

Voluntary testing units

There is a VTU on Kennet House Unit which caters for twenty trusted young people in their final year of sentence. Berkshire Probation Service run an offending behaviour programme over a six-week period. Other pre-release programmes, which involve outside employers, are in place.

Overall findings

The appointment of a drugs counsellor from ACORN is an example of good practice. ACORN run a drop-in centre in the association room on one day a week for those on induction; this enables young offenders to receive advice and guidance.

The inspectors make several recommendations including that:

- all newly appointed staff should receive drug awareness training;
- efforts to reduce the supply of illegal drugs coming into the establishment are to be increased by providing a passive and active drug dog;
- the disgraceful health and hygiene conditions in the MDT suite are addressed;
- the drug strategy is revised following a comprehensive needs analysis;
- the regime on the VTU is formally evaluated to assess its impact on young prisoners.

HMP AND YOI PARC

Parc is the first prison to be contracted out and run by Securicor. It opened in November 1997 with a Certified Normal Accommodation of 800 and an occupational capacity of 920. It acts as a local prison catering for remand and sentenced adults, young offenders and juveniles, although at the time of the inspection it accommodated 648 sentenced prisoners and young offenders.

The main offence of 9.5 per cent of the prisoners is drug-related, although the percentage is lower (5.2 per cent) amongst YOIs and juveniles.

What prisoners said

A group of young offenders told the inspectors:

* prisoners on the enhanced wing and VTU have in-cell TV;
* drugs are freely available, particularly speed and heroin;
* there is access to counsellors on the VTU;
* remand prisoners are not eligible to go on the VTU.

A group of adult remand prisoners told the inspectors:

* there are no detoxification arrangements for those admitted with a drugs problem;
* drugs are more freely available than in some establishments.

What the Director said

He said that a positive culture exists amongst staff, unlike the position in some prison service establishments. His vision is to provide a safe environment, provide full employment for prisoners, address offending behaviour and run a successful commercial enterprise.

The Board of Visitors are concerned that drug-taking is a big problem. Although the two voluntary testing units opened ahead of schedule, they think that CCTV coverage in the visits room is inadequate.

The drugs strategy

Many prisoners believe that drugs are freely available in the establishment with the exception of the long-term wings. They claim cannabis, heroin, crack, cocaine, speed, acid and ecstasy are easy to acquire. Most staff feel drugs misuse is a significant problem which could be tackled by introducing more CCTV in visits, using a drug dog, imposing stiffer punishments on those caught using class A drugs, and by improving staff training. Sixty-three per cent of staff have not received any Drugs Awareness training, although those that had stated the drugs training was 'very useful'.

The main route for drugs entering the prison is through personal visits. The CCTV system in the visits area is fairly basic, but there are plans to replace it with more sophisticated technology. There is a need for literature and more prominent signs to be displayed that warn visitors of the consequences of drug smuggling. The most pressing issue is to fund a passive drug dog to be present during visits. These plans are despite the fact that the bid submitted for CSR funding was unsuccessful.

The drug and alcohol strategy lacks central coordination and there is no evidence that a needs analysis has been carried out. The drugs strategy group have not met for nine months and the drugs strategy policy document is still in draft form and contains many inaccuracies.

During the inspection, a drug counsellor with responsibility for developing the prison's CARAT service was appointed to act as temporary drug strategy manager.

The inspectors feel there is scope for confusion and conflict over the roles and responsibilities of the wing managers and the drug strategy manager, who has operational responsibility for the VTU.

Reception
All new prisoners are screened for drug use by a nurse and where appropriate seen immediately by a doctor. Although there are no detoxification facilities, any prisoner who has been using methadone or opiates is offered a week-long symptom management course of lofexidine.

Health care
The clinical work undertaken with drug misusers needs to be properly evaluated and the findings published. There is a lack of written policies or procedures, and detoxification is not included in the treatment regime offered to prisoners identified with drug problems.

Throughcare
Two and a half drug workers were originally recruited to provide counselling services for prisoners. Since the introduction of the CARAT service and the setting up of VTUs, the focus of their role has changed to delivering groupwork. These staff are very committed and run high-quality groups which are valued by staff and prisoners.

The head of sentence planning is responsible for throughcare, including oversight of sentence management. Completed sentence plans are of good quality and contain realistic targets based on an individual needs analysis. Many sentence plans are not being completed which adversely affects short-term prisoners and young offenders. In the previous month, for instance, 55 sentence plans were not compiled.

The current target is to produce 1000 hours of groups per week. This is not realistic and cannot be achieved if accredited prison programmes are to be provided. Research has demonstrated that accredited prison programmes are effective in addressing offending behaviour. A criminogenic needs analysis should be conducted in the South Wales cluster of prisons to assess the level of offending behaviour work that needs addressing.

A psychologist should be recruited and existing groups phased out in favour of providing the Enhanced Thinking Skills and Reasoning and Rehabilitation programmes.

MDT
Ten per cent of the prisoner population are tested each month in accordance with Prison Service policy. The percentage of positive random tests is 41 per cent, which is mainly for cannabis and other class B drugs. These results support the belief that drugs are widely available and endemic in the South Wales catchment area.

Voluntary testing units
Two VTUs have been set up which cater for up to 88 prisoners on each unit. These units, which are segregated from the rest of the prison, cater for young offenders and

adult convicted prisoners. The treatment programme is well received by prisoners on the unit and consists of wing-based group meetings. Voluntary testing is carried out on the units using 'dip and read' testing.

Overall findings

The inspectors recommend the Drug and Alcohol Strategy Team reconvene, update the written drug strategy document, and conduct a comprehensive needs analysis of drug misuse in the establishment.

The inspectors also suggest that:

- further measures are introduced to discourage visitors from bringing drugs into Parc;
- a passive drug dog is present on visits;
- health care services are reviewed to ensure compliance with Prison Service standards on 'Clinical Services for Substance Misusers';
- the roles of the Drugs Strategy Manager and Wing Manager are clarified;
- a user-friendly brochure on drug issues is produced.

HMP EXETER

HMP Exeter is a Victorian local prison with a population of 476. The prisoners are accommodated in four wings and include adult remand and sentenced prisoners, eighteen lifers, 48 vulnerable prisoners, a wing of 71 young offenders and eight juveniles (between 16 and 18 years).

Remand prisoners make up 17.5 per cent of the population, with a further 44 per cent convicted but not sentenced. Ten per cent of the prisoners had a main offence that was drug-related.

What prisoners said

A group of young prisoners told the inspectors:

- half the prisoners on the wings were using drugs;
- nearly one third admitted taking drugs whilst at HMP Exeter;
- the drugs they took were amphetamines, cannabis, annitripilinex and ecstasy.

A group of convicted adult prisoners told the inspectors:

- large numbers of prisoners are placed on closed visits;
- health care services are very poor;
- mentally ill prisoners receive no help;
- there is a plentiful supply of heroin in the prison.

A group of adult remand prisoners told the inspectors:

• prisoners are placed on closed visits for petty reasons;
• holding a conversation is very difficult on closed visits due to the very thick glass.

The drugs strategy

HMP Exeter has published a comprehensive drugs strategy which was last updated in March 1998. It needs revising to take account of the additional services which are to be introduced as a result of CSR funding.

The drugs strategy group meet every two months and meetings are chaired by a senior governor grade. The group includes representatives from all relevant departments and service providers. It needs to become far more proactive and conduct a comprehensive needs analysis, collect and assess data, develop services more effectively and monitor the work of existing service providers.

The establishment is using CCTV successfully on visits. The absence of a passive drug dog and handler is being addressed with CSR funding, but staff shortages mean the searching programme is falling behind. At times, special searches are not able to be carried out in response to security intelligence received.

The inspectors feel the drugs strategy is in the early stages of development and CSR funding will help HMP Exeter develop a range of services for drug misusers.

Reception
Good reception procedures are in place and carried out by a group of cheerful and enthusiastic staff. All new receptions are seen by a nurse and the medical officer whilst in reception, and within a reasonable timespan.

Health care
Health care staff assess all new receptions for drug use and offer two detoxification treatment programmes. One uses diazepam for benzodiazepine detoxification; the other uses lofexidine to control the side effects of opioid withdrawal. Patients with complicated problems are admitted to the hospital for treatment; with simpler cases, they are seen on an out-patient basis. The supervision of patients receiving detoxification treatment is inadequate and does not meet the Department of Health guidelines on clinical management, because the withdrawal symptoms of patients are not monitored properly. The health care centre provides advice and guidance on matters relating to HIV and hepatitis, including testing and immunization services. Concern was expressed that the lack of information available about drug services in the prison is responsible for the low number of self-referrals for these services.

Throughcare
The Exeter Drugs Project, funded by the local health authority, offers some of the best treatment for substance abusers in the country. They assess the needs of prisoners and offer individual counselling, as well as running groups in partnership with the Probation Service. This service is to be absorbed into the new CARAT contract and,

as a consequence, will not receive any additional funding. Some prison staff, in partnership with NACRO (National Association for the Care and Resettlement of Offenders), are providing a drug awareness group to around 70 per cent of the young prisoners in the course of a year. Uncertainty remains about whether sufficient staff resources will be available in the future to permit this initiative to continue.

MDT
MDT is carried out in an extremely well designed and equipped MDT suite and all the staff have received appropriate MDT training. During the past twelve months, the level of testing has fallen below the required standard (10 per cent of the population), falling to 5.9 per cent during 1998–9, leading to the MDT staff becoming disheartened.

The percentage of positive random tests in the previous twelve months was 27.9 per cent and the number of 'on suspicion' tests that proved positive was 60 per cent. The most commonly detected drugs were cannabis, followed by opiates and benzo-diazepines.

A major failing was an inability to lay disciplinary charges for MDT positive results within the required 48 hour deadline of the results being received from the laboratory. This had occurred thirteen times in the first four months of 1999, meaning that 29 per cent of drug users were escaping punishment.

Voluntary testing units
There is no VTU at HMP Exeter at present. There are plans to develop a facility using CSR funding and officers are currently being recruited to undertake voluntary testing.

Overall findings

The inspectors were aware that additional funding is being provided so that drug programmes and offending behaviour groups, based on a cognitive skills approach, can be provided. They believe the culture at HMP Exeter needs to change and that staff must stop perceiving the prison as a transit camp; it needs to be seen as an establishment that gives high priority to effectively preparing prisoners for release, with the emphasis placed on running offending behaviour courses and helping those with drug problems.

The inspectors make several recommendations including the following:

- a passive drugs dog and handler should be provided;
- MDT testing should be improved;
- the drug strategy group should collate and evaluate all available data;
- the drug strategy group should produce an information leaflet that explains to new receptions what drug services are available;
- the level of CARAT services provided should be discussed with the local Drug Action Team;
- the arrangements for searching prisoners and visitors should be improved;
- a needs analysis of drug misuse should be conducted;
- some form of pre-release preparation should be provided for all discharges.

HMP AND YOI BULLWOOD HALL

Bullwood Hall is a Young Offender Institution and closed prison for women and has a CNA of 140. At the time of the inspection there were 131 prisoners of which seventeen were juveniles (those between the ages of 15 and 17), and 41 young offenders (those between the ages of 18 and 20). A 'ready-to-use' unit (RTU) is being made ready to provide accommodation for a further 40 female prisoners.

The main offence of 25.95 per cent of the women is drug-related.

The drugs strategy

The inspectors make no reference to the drug strategy since they concentrate on following up the recommendations they made on an earlier inspection in May 1997.

A CCTV system is in place in the visits room where pre-booked visits take place. However, rub-down searches still take place in a passageway outside the visits room and strip searches around the corner in the same area.

Reception

Although some needs are identified on reception and through the sentence management process, no comprehensive needs analysis is undertaken. This should be addressed as a priority and an information technology database set up to coordinate this information.

Health care

Some women continue to use other prisoners' medication without authority, although the position is improving. Closer liaison between health care staff and those responsible for drug testing should be developed.

Throughcare

There is little in the way of treatment to offer women who fail drug tests. Anger management courses no longer run and there are no plans to reintroduce pre-release courses.

CSR funding could help the development of a range of drug rehabilitation programmes in the three Kent prisons. Bullwood Hall is planning to deliver accredited Enhanced Thinking Skills courses and groupwork programmes based on the criminogenic needs of the women.

Existing treatment programmes are poor; the drug counsellor is no longer providing a counselling service and there are no accredited offending behaviour courses. The only courses available are provided through the Education Department.

MDT

MDT testing is frequently cancelled which means that agreed targets – 5 per cent random testing and 10 per cent targeted testing – are not being achieved. Sufficient trained staff are available to carry out drug tests but time to conduct the tests is not being provided.

Voluntary testing units
There is no voluntary testing unit or evidence of voluntary testing taking place.

Overall findings

Bullwood Hall is on the list of establishments identified by the Prison Service as needing closer managerial attention. However, it is making progress. Sentence planning is being hampered by the absence of any accredited offending behaviour courses. Mandatory drug testing targets can only be achieved if sufficient time is allocated to this task. Rub-down searches should not be carried out in a passageway and graffiti should be removed from the search area.

HMP PRESTON

HMP Preston is a Victorian inner-city local prison with a population of 640, who are accommodated on five wings. Thirty-five per cent of the population are remand prisoners and a further 7.9 per cent are convicted but not sentenced.

The main offence of 12.7 per cent of the prisoners is drug-related.

What prisoners said

A group of convicted prisoners told the inspectors:

- those undergoing detoxification have to mix with other prisoners;
- there are no personal officers;
- prisoners have their own drug officer.

A group of remand prisoners told the inspectors:

- they never see a probation officer;
- they feel safe because there is no bullying in the establishment;
- there are few drugs at HMP Preston.

The drugs strategy

There is a drugs strategy committee which is chaired by a governor grade and meets monthly. The drug strategy is effectively coordinated and all departments and relevant agencies are represented. No needs analysis of the scale of the drugs problem or the extent of drug misuse within the prison has been conducted.

The prison has difficulty controlling the supply of illegal drugs due to the high turnover of prisoners. The poor layout in the visits room coupled with a significant amount of overcrowding makes it difficult to prevent drug trafficking.

Any prisoner placed on closed visits has his case reviewed each month. Those considered suitable for removal are placed on non-contact visits for a further month; this is a practice the inspectors do not endorse.

The state of disrepair and appalling lack of cleanliness on closed visits is a cause for concern. The inspectors also found closed visits are being reduced to fifteen minutes, half the official allowance.

The building where visits are held makes it difficult for passive drug dogs to operate effectively, whilst the lack of CCTV coverage in the visits room adds to the problems facing staff. A bid for CCTV, under CSR funding, has been provisionally approved.

The inspectors feel HMP Preston is developing a positive response to drug issues, especially since limited resources are available to tackle the problem. Some staff view this proactive approach to tackling drug misuse as a concession to prisoners, but the majority of staff embrace an innovative approach to tackling drug issues.

Reception

The inspectors consider the conditions in reception fail spectacularly to meet laid-down standards due to poor state of repair and non-compliance with Prison Service Operating Standards.

New receptions arrive at Preston on six days a week between 1315 and 2100 hours and are seen by a nurse. Whilst on induction they are interviewed about their drug use and informed about drug services available in the establishment. There is scope to improve the dissemination of information by presenting this material in an attractive booklet.

Prisoners undergoing detoxification are in need of a more comprehensive induction programme than is currently provided.

Health care

Those prisoners identified as needing detoxification provide a urine sample and are offered assessment the following day. The treatment programme comprises seven to ten days of dihydrocodeine, in conjunction with tranquillizers to control the symptoms.

Methadone is not being prescribed by the senior medical officer; this contravenes the health care standard guidelines issue by the Prison Service. The inspectors recommend that 'the clinical judgement for prescribing is reassessed'.

Throughcare

The throughcare committee hold meetings quarterly. Although help for drug misusers is provided together with a good bail information scheme, insufficient help is available to address housing, unemployment and resettlement needs.

All residential wings have their own drug key worker who is specially selected and receives a minimum of three days' training. Their commitment and enthusiasm is appreciated by prisoners and their contribution is shortly to be complemented by workers through the CARAT service.

The Probation Department offer a range of programmes in partnership with prison officers. They include a basic Drug Awareness course and a more advanced Drug and Offending Behaviour course. In addition, probation officers offer Anger Management and Alcohol Awareness courses.

All agencies working in the establishment work effectively together to provide services to drug users. The Education Department offers Drug Awareness classes and the PE Department makes individual need assessments and provides programmes for drug users. A close working relationship exists with the Probation Department who receives referrals for their courses from other departments. Although none of the courses offered are accredited, there are plans to validate existing non-accredited courses.

A drugs worker is employed who provides an impressive service. The service is funded jointly by a voluntary drugs agency and the local health trust. Prison officers provide assessment and ongoing support to many of the prisoners passing through HMP Preston with an identifiable drug dependency problem.

MDT

MDT is conducted in a fully equipped and well designed dedicated suite by a group of prison officers. The number of MDT tests carried out is only 50 per cent of the laid-down national standard, with 405 tests completed in 1998–9 compared to the target figure of 810. The rate of positive tests over this twelve-month period is 26 per cent. However, this figure is unreliable due to the limited number of random tests taking place.

Every prisoner who has an MDT is dealt with fairly and humanely by well trained, experienced prison officers. MDT staff support the overall drug strategy and routinely offer information about drug services available within the establishment to prisoners. The governorial team take a constructive approach with those prisoners who appear on internal disciplinary charges for drug offences.

Voluntary testing units

Although there is no VTU or drug-free area at Preston, a voluntary testing programme is offered to prisoners involved in probation run programmes.

Comprehensive Spending Review funding has already been allocated to recruit staff for a drug dependency unit to be based on C1 landing. It will offer a three-week rolling detoxification programme for up to 60 prisoners. Once established, voluntary testing can be extended to all prisoners resident on C Wing.

Overall findings

Many aspects of the drug strategy at HMP Preston are positive, largely because good relationships exist between different disciplines and agencies involved in service delivery.

The inspectors made several recommendations which include identifying a need to:

- examine the scale of the drug problem within HMP Preston and conduct a needs analysis;
- incorporate performance targets into service level agreements with other agencies;
- install CCTV in the visits area;

- revise the current practice of reviewing closed visits;
- increase the level of MDT that is taking place;
- improve the use and deployment of drug dogs;
- produce an information booklet for drug users;
- reassess prescribing practice and the non-use of methadone.

HMYOI HATFIELD

Hatfield is an open establishment which caters for 180 prisoners aged between 18 and 21. It comprises three house units, although one unit is temporarily closed due to a lack of prisoners available for transfer from secure YOIs.

The main offence of 4.1 per cent of the prisoners is drug-related.

What prisoners said

A group of prisoners told the inspectors:

- Mandatory drug testing takes place regularly;
- anyone found using opiates is returned to closed conditions;
- prisoners failing a drugs test are likely to be placed on the basic regime;
- the personal officer scheme works well and is appreciated by the prisoners.

The drugs strategy

The drug strategy team includes representation from each department and meets biannually, although the drugs strategy policy document calls for regular quarterly meetings. The policy document needs updating because recent developments concerning CARAT services and CSR funding have been omitted.

A voluntary agency, the Substance Abuse Referral Unit (SARU), provides a specialist part-time drug worker and performs a valuable service. Lengthy waiting lists continue to be a problem because no cover is provided for annual leave or sickness.

Hatfield does not have its own passive or active drug dog, but receives occasional assistance from neighbouring establishments.

An innovative idea is a peripatetic puppet theatre which runs sessions on drug issues for up to 50 prisoners each visit.

Reception

Health care staff see new receptions and question them about their drug use. Where appropriate they are referred to the specialist drug worker. A profile of previous drug use is non-existent because no one collates this information.

The induction programme is criticized for spending insufficient time on drug misuse issues because the original plan for a specific drug awareness session has been replaced by an input on HIV/AIDS.

Health care
No needs assessment of health care services has been conducted and there is minimal involvement by health care staff in helping drug misusers. The inspectors' view is that health care services should be contributing to the induction programme, pre-release courses and the overall drug strategy.

Throughcare
Despite the absence of a proper needs analysis, personal officers contribute fully to the sentence management process.

Prison officers run an excellent pre-release course catering for prisoners during the final week of their sentence. Although it is not an accredited course, formal feedback sessions take place and it is described as a stimulating and helpful experience.

Offending behaviour groups have been discontinued, largely because there is a belief that non-accredited courses are counter-productive. Hatfield originally acted as a pilot establishment for the substance abuse module, which is part of the Young Offender Treatment Programme (YOTP), and ran three groups. These substance abuse groups were discontinued after they failed to meet the required standard for accreditation.

MDT
MDT is conducted to a high standard in a discrete suite and random drug testing takes place regularly. In the previous twelve months, 9.1 per cent of the population were tested and 16.2 per cent tested positive.

The MDT coordinator takes responsibility for collating and processing security information reports (SIRs) involving staff effectively. Regular drug intelligence is received at the rate of 20 to 30 SIRs each month. The quality of intelligence allows effective preventative action to be taken against drug dealers and those suspected of using drugs.

Voluntary testing units
The drug strategy action plan intends that voluntary drug testing should be available to all prisoners on the enhanced wing. CSR funding is being provided to set up a VTU and recruit an additional drug worker.

Overall findings

Good intelligence systems at Hatfield have allowed staff to keep the drug problem under control despite limited resources. Drug services could be improved by providing relapse prevention support, and cognitive and motivational groupwork.

The inspectors make the following specific recommendations:

- the drug strategy team should meet more frequently;
- the drug strategy policy document needs updating;
- information about the level of drug misuse should be collected when prisoners are on induction;

- more time needs spending on drug awareness issues during the induction period;
- health care staff should provide an input to the induction programme, pre-release courses and drug initiatives;
- drug services need to address the specific needs of the 18 to 21 year olds.

HMP WAYLAND

Wayland is a modern, purpose-built category C training prison which opened in 1985 with four wings and now has six wings. It has a CNA of 620 and an occupational capacity of 648.

What prisoners said

A group of prisoners told the inspectors that:

- Offending Behaviour groups are provided for the prisoners in the Vulnerable Prisoner Unit (VPU);
- prisoners on ordinary location are not given sufficient access to practical help.

What the Governor said

The Governor feels the Security Department are making positive progress in tackling drugs, particularly since the arrival of drug dogs and the introduction of a better security information system.

The Governor fully supports the introduction of accredited Offending Behaviour programmes but is concerned the existing resettlement programmes for short-sentenced prisoners is not neglected.

The drugs strategy

The inspectors do not specifically refer to the drug strategy as their primary focus is on progress made in implementing recommendations from the previous inspection conducted in 1995 and published in April 1996.

There is a coherent drugs strategy policy which is clearly understood by all staff and results in integrated care for prisoners. Each wing has drug liaison officers who are allocated sufficient time to carry out their duties.

Reception
A good induction programme is offered to all prisoners. Lifers and vulnerable prisoners have a separate programme. A comprehensive needs assessment is necessary which should be integrated into the sentence management process. There is scope to rationalize and reduce the number of compacts in use.

Health care
Health care staff identify prisoners on reception who have not received hepatitis B immunization and offer them the service.

Throughcare
A number of excellent groups are taking place throughout the prison including an anger management programme. Wayland needs to adopt an integrated approach which is based on a needs assessment related to their offending behaviour. There is no evaluation of non-accredited groups taking place, and the inspectors consider all groups should be based on recognized theory and fully evaluated.

The sentence management unit is impressive and is staffed by a multi-disciplinary team. They deliver non-accredited courses and the Enhanced Thinking Skills course with enthusiasm.

MDT
Monthly statistics on the extent and type of drug-taking at Wayland are collated and studied locally by the Security Committee and as part of the drug strategy.

Voluntary testing units
The inspectors highlight the good work being done on the drug rehabilitation unit (DRU), where they describe the quality of care being offered to prisoners as exceptional. The structure and organization of the DRU has been revised and it acts as a national resource for the Prison Service, offering an impressive standard of care to prisoners.

Overall findings
The inspectors conclude by saying that 'Wayland is a thoroughly healthy prison'. They are extremely impressed with the work undertaken in the drug rehabilitation unit which they consider to be exceptional. They recommend further investment in a treatment manager, a nurse, psychological support and more throughcare services.

They make several other recommendations:

- all groupwork should be evaluated;
- research should be conducted into prisoners' needs;
- Offending Behaviour programmes, including booster programmes, should be geared to prisoners' identified needs;
- health education should be included in the induction programme.

HMP AND HMYOI HOLLESLEY BAY COLONY

Hollesley Bay holds a mixture of adults and young offenders. At the time of the inspection, 321 prisoners were accommodated in five units. Two units are based in Warren Hill, the site of the original YOI, where 136 young adults and 44 juveniles reside. Adult prisoners (including some lifers) are held in open conditions on Cosford and Wilforde units, whilst Stowe unit provides open conditions for young offenders.

The number of prisoners who have a main offence which is drug-related is not disclosed in the inspection report.

The drugs strategy

The inspectors recognize the establishment have produced a drug strategy and are in the process of implementing it. Problems remain in preventing drugs entering the establishment despite the acquisition of a drug dog to combat trafficking.

When Warren Hill opened in 1982, it was a closed establishment for young offenders consisting of four units. Two units are being converted into juvenile units in line with the requirements of the Youth Justice Board, whilst the remaining units continue to hold adults. There are plans to turn one unit into a drug rehabilitation unit and use the other as a voluntary testing unit.

Reception
The induction programme is superficial with insufficient information being provided to young people on first reception into custody. However, compacts have been introduced which set out the responsibilities of both staff and prisoners.

Health care
There is a real need for a qualified psychiatric nurse to screen all young offenders on reception to identify any of them exhibiting signs of severe mental or emotional problems.

A needs assessment should identify substance misusers and address those with drug problems.

Throughcare
A needs analysis should identify a range of Offending Behaviour courses including booster courses for short-term prisoners.

The Education Department have previously run pre-release courses. These have been discontinued and pre-release courses are no longer available to young adults.

Drug awareness and addiction groups take place on a regular basis, and cater for the needs of all prisoners and young offenders. These courses need to be evaluated and accredited Offending Behaviour groups introduced.

MDT
No information is available on random testing.

Voluntary testing units
There are plans to have a VTU based in one of the units at Warren Hill.

Overall findings

The inspectors made the following recommendations:

- all new arrivals should be screened by a psychiatric nurse;
- accredited Offending Behaviour groups should be introduced;
- Gipping unit should be developed as a drug rehabilitation unit;
- a voluntary testing unit should be introduced.

CHAPTER 10

Planning for the Future

ASSESSING CURRENT PERFORMANCE

The HMCIP have inspected a cross section of establishments during 1999 and the overall picture emerging is that most prisons are making headway towards having in place an effective drugs strategy.

The HMCIP findings show that, a year after the launch of the drugs strategy, measurable progress is taking place. Most establishments appear to be developing comprehensive plans using Comprehensive Spending Funding Review, and are setting up voluntary testing units, improving their security detection measures and mandatory drug testing performance, and making plans to deliver accredited Offending Behaviour programmes.

There is little evidence that much progress has occurred in establishments catering for young offenders. This was a worrying finding for, given the evidence about the scale of drug use amongst young people in the community, the importance of targeting young offenders and making early interventions should be self evident. Since April 2000 the Juvenile Estate has been established which should address these problems.

Performance ratings

The table that follows assesses the performance of establishments based on areas the inspectors identified as important in their reports. The criteria used to assess key aspects of service delivery in each establishment is in compliance with policy standards. Performance is rated as GOOD, ACCEPTABLE or DEFICIENT, with three points allocated to a function rated Good, two to an Acceptable marking, and one point where a deficiency is highlighted.

An overall score of eighteen means that the policy 'Tackling Drugs in Prison' has been fully implemented and high standards are being maintained.

An overall score of twelve and above indicates good progress is being made to meet the requirements of the drugs policy, and the independent Chief Inspector of Prisons appears to be satisfied on balance with the progress achieved.

The overall ratings show HMP Bristol to be a model of good practice. On the other hand, HMYOI Huntercombe and HMP and YOI Bullwood Hall appear to have made little progress towards tackling drug misuse in their establishments. However, it

Table 3: Overall rating assessment

	Drugs strategy	Reception	Health care	Throughcare	MDT	VTU	Overall score
HMP Liverpool	Acceptable	Acceptable	Deficient	Good	Good	Deficient	12
HMP Wymott	Deficient	Good	Deficient	Good	Good	Deficient	12
HMP Wormwood Scrubs	Acceptable	Deficient	Acceptable	Acceptable	Acceptable	Good	12
HMYOI Huntercombe	Deficient	Deficient	Deficient	Acceptable	Deficient	Deficient	7
HMP Highdown	Deficient	Deficient	Deficient	Acceptable	Deficient	Acceptable	8
HMP Bristol	Good	Good	Good	Good	Good	Good	18
HMP and RC Reading	Acceptable	Good	Acceptable	Acceptable	Deficient	Good	13
HMP Parc	Acceptable	Good	Deficient	Acceptable	Acceptable	Good	13
HMP Exeter	Acceptable	Good	Acceptable	Good	Deficient	Deficient	12
HMP and YOI Bullwood Hall	Deficient	Acceptable	Deficient	Deficient	Deficient	Deficient	7
HMP Preston	Acceptable	Deficient	Acceptable	Good	Good	Acceptable	13
HMYOI Hatfield	Acceptable	Deficient	Deficient	Acceptable	Good	Deficient	10
HMP Wayland	Acceptable	Acceptable	Acceptable	Good	Good	Good	15
HMP and HMYOI Hollesley Bay Colony	Acceptable	Acceptable	Deficient	Acceptable	Deficient	Deficient	9

should be borne in mind that CARAT treatment services had not yet been introduced at this stage in the establishments inspected.

ANALYSING COMPARATIVE DATA

This analysis of comparative data, based on the HMCIP inspection reports, takes the form of a league table which ranks the overall performance of fourteen establishments appearing in this sample under two headings. The first heading Prisons covers establishments holding male adult prisoners, the second heading YOIs covers establishments holding young offenders under the age of 21.

Table 4: League tables

Best		Best	
Prisons	Overall score	*YOIs*	Overall score
1. Bristol	18	1. Reading	13
2. Wayland	15	2. Hatfield	10
3 = Parc	13	3. Hollesley Bay Colony	9
3 = Preston	13	4 = Huntercombe	7
5 = Liverpool	12	4 = Bullwood Hall (female)	7
5 = Wymott	12		
5 = Wormwood Scrubs	12		
5 = Exeter	12		
9. Highdown	8		

Table 5: Numerical overall rating assessment

	Drugs strategy	Reception	Health care	Throughcare	MDT	VTU	Score	Ranking
Liverpool	2	2	1	3	3	1	12	6 =
Wymott	1	3	1	3	3	1	12	6 =
Wormwood Scrubs	2	1	2	2	2	3	12	6 =
Huntercombe	1	1	1	2	1	1	7	13 =
Highdown	1	1	1	2	1	2	8	12
Bristol	3	3	3	3	3	3	18	1
Reading	2	3	2	2	1	3	13	3 =
Parc	2	3	1	2	2	3	13	3 =
Exeter	2	3	2	3	1	1	12	6 =
Bullwood Hall	1	2	1	1	1	1	7	13 =
Preston	2	1	2	3	3	2	13	3 =
Hatfield	2	1	1	2	3	1	10	10
Wayland	2	2	2	3	3	3	15	2
Hollesley Bay	2	2	1	2	1	1	9	11

3 = Good, 2 = Acceptable, 1 = Deficient

The most noticeable conclusion that emerges from these league tables is that, in the opinion of HMCIP inspectors, most prisons examined are significantly better than those establishments catering for young offenders.

This finding is interesting in the context that 'helping young people resist drug misuse in order to achieve their full potential in society' is the first aim in the Government's national ten-year strategy to 'Tackling Drugs To Build a Better Britain'. On the reasonable assumption that this is a representative sample and the HMCIP inspectors are consistent in the criteria they apply, a number of questions are reasonable to pose:

- Is greater priority being given to addressing drug issues in establishments holding adult male prisoners?
- Do the widely differing levels of practice reflect historically different baselines?
- Is the strategy being implemented consistently across the country?
- Does the way funding is allocated across the prison estate need to be reviewed?
- Is there an argument for injecting funding into establishments holding young offenders to redress this imbalance?
- Are Governors given too much discretion about setting priorities?

The drugs strategy

The following establishments examined by the inspectors in 1999 are implementing the 'Tackling Drugs in Prison' policy. They have in place a drugs strategy team or committee to identify the scale of the problem locally, and have devised strategies to tackle the supply of drugs, reduce the demand for them, provide effective treatment opportunities and make resources available to combat drugs effectively.

Prisons	*YOIs*
HMP Bristol	HMYOI and RC Reading
HMP Liverpool	HMYOI Hatfield
HMP Wormwood Scrubs	HMP and HMYOI Hollesley Bay Colony
HMP Parc	
HMP Exeter	
HMP Preston	
HMP Wayland	
7 out of 9 prisons conform	3 out of 5 YOIs conform
78 per cent compliance	60 per cent compliance

Reception

The following establishments examined by the inspectors in 1999 have reception procedures which facilitate the drugs strategy. They use a range of staff to identify and address drug misuse on first reception into custody and provide a comprehensive induction programme.

Prisons	*YOIs*
HMP Wymott	HMP and RC Reading
HMP Bristol	HMP and YOI Bullwood Hall
HMP Parc	HMP and HMYOI Hollesley Bay Colony
HMP Exeter	
HMP Liverpool	
HMP Wayland	
6 out of 9 prisons conform	3 out of 5 YOIs conform
67 per cent compliance	60 per cent compliance

Health care

Only a minority of establishments inspected in 1999 have health care procedures in place which meet the standards set out in the drugs strategy. These include health care screening, detoxification facilities in a local prison, or providing appropriate levels of care to those with a drug problem. The Healthcare Standard has been revised and is awaiting publication.

Prisons	*YOIs*
HMP Bristol	HMYOI and RC Reading
HMP Wormwood Scrubs	
HMP Exeter	
HMP Preston	
HMP Wayland	
5 out of 9 prisons conform	1 out of 5 YOIs conform
56 per cent compliance	20 per cent compliance

Throughcare

Most establishments provide a comprehensive throughcare service which includes providing a range of groups for those who need help addressing their drug problem. Although the groups offered are not normally accredited programmes, they are, in the view of the inspectors, consistent with the drugs strategy.

Prisons	*YOIs*
HMP Liverpool	HMYOI Huntercombe
HMP Wymott	HMYOI and RC Reading
HMP Bristol	HMYOI Hatfield
HMP Exeter	HMP and HMYOI Hollesley Bay Colony
HMP Preston	
HMP Wayland	
HMP Wormwood Scrubs	
HMP Highdown	
HMP Parc	
9 out of 9 prisons conform	4 out of 5 YOIs conform
100 per cent compliance	80 per cent compliance

Mandatory drug testing

The following establishments examined by the inspectors in 1999 conduct mandatory drug testing to a standard consistent with the drugs strategy.

Prisons	*YOIs*
HMP Liverpool	HMYOI Hatfield
HMP Wymott	
HMP Bristol	
HMP Preston	
HMP Wayland	
HMP Wormwood Scrubs	
HMP Parc	
7 out of 9 prisons conform	1 out of 5 YOIs conform
78 per cent compliance	20 per cent compliance

Voluntary testing unit

The following establishments inspected in 1999 have set up a voluntary testing unit, or offer voluntary testing facilities to inmates to a standard which in the inspectors' view complies with the requirements of the drugs strategy.

Prisons	*YOIs*
HMP Wormwood Scrubs	HMYOI and RC Reading
HMP Bristol	
HMP Parc	
HMP Wayland	
HMP Highdown	
HMP Preston	
6 out of 9 prisons conform	1 out of 5 YOIs conform
67 per cent compliance	20 per cent compliance

FORWARD PLANNING

'Tackling Drugs in Prison' is a relatively new strategy (May 1998) which builds on the lessons and good practice established in the earlier policy document 'Drug Misuse in Prison' (April 1995).

The latest policy initiative, 'Tackling Drugs to Build a Better Britain', has been supported by a considerable amount of additional funding following the Comprehensive Spending Review. The amount allocated to the Prison Service was £76 million spread over three years (1999 to 2002) which is additional to the baseline level of £9 million per annum which is continuing.

It would be premature to judge the success of this policy initiative at this early stage. The criteria for success is to reduce the overall level of offending and assess to what extent it is cost-effective. Many observers would conclude that it is a worthwhile investment if it reduces human misery to drug abusers and their relatives, makes some impact on reconviction rates and, as a consequence, reduces the overall number of victims in society.

There are encouraging signs of progress, because where the drugs strategy is fully operational, as at HMP Bristol, the impact is considerable. Although the HMCIP reports highlight that there is still much to be achieved, a recurring theme in the reports is that CSR funding has been allocated and the resources are in the process of being acquired. In this sense the story is 'to be continued'. The policy is being resourced and implementation is taking place across the prison estate.

The Home Affairs Committee report 'Drugs and Prisons' (November 1999) concludes (in paragraph 36) that the Prison Service has taken steps in the right direction: 'The new strategy takes forward in a positive and considered way the initiatives developed in earlier years and provides a platform for progress towards making a period of imprisonment an opportunity for reducing offenders' involvement with drugs.'

Undoubtedly concerns exist, which should not be discounted, about the scale of unmet need that CARAT service assessments are now identifying in some establishments. Other concerns relate to the ability of the Prison Service to obtain sufficient resources from the Treasury to provide the necessary range of treatment services within penal establishments and the supporting throughcare services in the prisons and community. However, these anxieties are dwarfed by the realization that community-based drug services are being overwhelmed by demand. Some authorities have been unwilling to acknowledge their responsibilities to provide for the ongoing needs of ex-offenders, whilst others are actively discriminating against them.

Notwithstanding these reservations, 'Tackling Drugs in Prison' is probably the most significant policy development since the Woolf Report and is a major step forward towards the ultimate goal to reduce offending by:

- providing 'decent conditions to prisoners' (the abolition of slopping out);
- treating prisoners fairly and 'looking after them with humanity' (the IEPS Scheme and request/complaint system);
- helping 'them live law-abiding and useful lives in custody and after release' (the drugs strategy).

'Tackling Drugs in Prison' requires the adoption of a holistic approach to those with drug problems within establishments by incorporating all of the following elements:

- joint working with the Probation Service on practice issues such as joint risk assessments, joint programme accreditation and improving collaboration by the shared use of resources;
- developing an enterprise culture in prisons through education, PE and meaningful work;
- providing accredited Offending Behaviour programmes which are targeted on those most likely to benefit from them;

- providing basic drug treatment services in all establishments;
- providing specialist drugs treatment services on an area and national basis;
- linking CARAT services in a systematic way to the criminal justice system and the process of seamless throughcare, which includes addressing accommodation and employment needs;
- catering for those with special needs, such as severely personality disordered offenders and those with mental health problems;
- providing high-quality drug education programmes for juveniles and young offenders;
- meeting the needs of women and ethnic minorities.

Future developments

The Prison Service is developing a joint accreditation panel with responsibility for accrediting Offending Behaviour programmes for both the Prison Service and Probation Service.

The Prison Service currently provides two accredited Living Skills programmes: Reasoning and Rehabilitation programme (35 sessions); and Enhanced Thinking Skills (20 sessions).

A number of additional accredited programmes are under development. These will address offending behaviour and cater for the needs of those with drug problems:

- Adult Acquisitive Offender programme;
- Anger and Emotion management;
- Cognitive and Self-Change programme;
- Dialectical Behavioural therapy;
- Drug programmes;
- Young Offender Treatment programmes.

Staff Training

PDM Consulting Ltd recently undertook a review of prison-based drug treatment and rehabilitation services and concluded that staff running programmes lacked knowledge and that drug awareness levels amongst prison officers were poor.

During summer 1999, the Drugs Strategy Unit in Prison Service headquarters initiated a Training Needs Analysis. The objectives were:

- to review what is currently being provided;
- to identify what training is needed to address this skills deficiency;
- to cost the resulting proposals.

The scope of the review is wide-ranging and focuses on the training needs of staff involved in providing the following services:

- mandatory drug testing;
- voluntary testing units;

- CARAT services;
- rehabilitation programmes and therapeutic communities;
- detoxification;
- health care;
- security intelligence.

The review will agree the minimum standard of drug awareness needed by the whole range of staff who work in penal establishments and identify what competencies are necessary to deliver CARAT services and work effectively in therapeutic communities.

The methodology adopted involves using questionnaires, visiting establishments and training providers, and analysing existing training outcomes.

The final report is due for publication during 2000 and is expected to identify there is scope for greater consistency in training provision based on core competencies and a core curriculum at various levels. It is expected to provide a central framework for Areas to plan to meet their training needs within their own areas.

THE INTERNATIONAL DIMENSION

Research carried out in the USA and UK indicates that between 20 and 50 per cent of illicit drug use is financed by crime. Most studies show that drug abuse usually occurs during adolescence or young adulthood, but illegal use declines from the late twenties onwards. The evidence demonstrates that the earlier drug misuse begins, the more likely it is to become problematic and habit forming.

Injecting drugs is a high risk activity because of the possibility of becoming infected with HIV/AIDS due to using contaminated injection equipment. Estimates of the numbers infected are between 280 and 560 million worldwide, which is equivalent to 5–10 per cent of the world's population.

Injecting drugs is responsible for 100 to 200,000 deaths a year throughout the world. To put this figure in context, it should be compared to the deaths that result from legally available products such as alcohol and tobacco, which are significantly worse: alcohol-related deaths are $\frac{3}{4}$–1 million every year; and tobacco-related deaths exceed 3 million each year.

Table 6: The scale of drug abuse

Drug misusers	Users (millions)	Percentage of world population
Cannabis	140	2.5
Amphetamine-type stimulants	30	0.5
Cocaine	13	0.23
Heroin	8	0.14

DECRIMINALIZATION

Under the Misuse of Drugs Act 1971, drugs are divided into three classes which are defined as 'controlled drugs'. The act sets out maximum penalties for their unlawful possession:

- **Class A**
  Cocaine, crack, ecstasy, heroin, LSD, amphetamines (if prepared for injection) and cannabis oil.
  Maximum penalty: 7 years' imprisonment and/or a fine.
- **Class B**
  Cannabis, amphetamines.
  Maximum penalty: 5 years' imprisonment and/or a fine.
- **Class C**
  Rohypnol, temazepam.
  Maximum penalty: 5 years' imprisonment and/or a fine.

The issue of decriminalization is likely to be subject to intense public debate in the next few years. Recent studies have found that 40 per cent of the population has, or is experiencing, soft drugs on a regular basis and that 49 per cent of young people have taken cannabis. A survey that sought the views of young people revealed that 75 per cent of those under 21 think cannabis should be decriminalized.

Decriminalization means the Government keeps in place criminal penalties for supplying and distributing the drug, but allows individuals to have cannabis in possession for their own personal consumption.

Changing attitudes

Attitudes in this country towards the use of soft drugs have changed significantly during the past twenty years. It is normal practice for the police to caution those found in possession of small quantities of cannabis for their personal use, whereas in 1992 only 45 per cent received a caution. In 1981, it was extremely rare, and only 1 per cent received a caution.

The Home Affairs Committee examining 'The Work of the UK Anti-Drugs Coordinator' took evidence from Keith Hellawell on 30 March 1999 on the question of decriminalization. He told the Committee that the police are free to use their discretion to caution people and take action other than prosecuting people through the courts: 'We can deal with substances such as cannabis in a way that would be described as public acceptance, but within the framework of the criminal justice system.'

The committee were advised that the prevalence of cannabis use amongst school children is so widespread that it has become normal behaviour. The problem facing young people is that they are not 'with it' if they experiment with cannabis as their first drug – smoking dope is hardly rebellious or radical, and nor is it beating the system to be doing what has become the norm.

Hellawell is conscious that cannabis is the most widely used drug in this country and believes it can cause regular users significant problems, particularly if taken with alcohol, and lead to psychological problems.

He points out that in Holland cannabis is treated as an illegal substance, but citizens are exempt from prosecution, providing they use it for personal consumption. The Dutch are very liberal and allow their citizens to buy cannabis in the 'so-called cafes'. This drug tourism was causing disturbances in the vicinity of the cafes, so they have reduced the number of cafes and restricted the amount that can be purchased to take away from 30 grams to 5 grams.

The medical dimension

Cannabis has been used as a medicine in China, India, the Middle East and South America for centuries. European doctors have been familiar with its medicinal value for well over a thousand years. Even Queen Victoria used it in the nineteenth century to reduce her labour pains.

In 1995 the World Health Organization concluded that dronabinol, one of the active ingredients in cannabis, has medicinal value. Its therapeutic value is to combat nausea in patients undergoing chemotherapy for cancer. Since then the controls on prescribing dronabinol in the UK have been relaxed.

Many people claim that cannabis and cannabis derivatives have medicinal value. Beneficial effects are reported by those suffering with multiple sclerosis who experience a reduction in spasms and tremors; AIDS sufferers who find it improves their appetite; and those undergoing treatment for glaucoma.

A recent opinion poll revealed that 89 per cent of the population think cannabis should be made legal for medicinal purposes.

Keith Hellawell told the Home Affairs Committee he had visited a cannabis farm run by GW Chemicals who are looking at its use for medicinal reasons, and stated: 'If it can be proved (under the provisions of the World Health Organization) these substances are safe to take, then I would support their use for medicinal purposes.'

The Committee were told the next stage is to hold field trials on people with medical conditions which, if successful, could result in cannabis receiving certification.

The European dimension

A change in attitude towards using cannabis throughout Europe is clearly discernible, with a very relaxed approach taken towards possession of cannabis for personal consumption. Some European countries, notably the Netherlands and some parts of Germany, have condoned the possession of small quantities of cannabis for personal use over a number of years.

Most European countries have legislation which prohibits having drugs in possession. In practice, they tend to impose minimal penalties in respect of cannabis.

Austria   No proceedings are taken against anyone using cannabis for personal consumption.

Belgium	Personal users normally receive a suspended sentence.
Denmark	No proceedings are instituted if possession is for personal use.
Finland	Possession normally results in a fine.
France	The Justice Ministry advises against prosecuting offenders and recommends giving warnings.
Germany	Tolerates the possession of cannabis for personal use.
Greece	Possession of small quantities for personal use can result in a fine.
Ireland	Personal possession can lead to a fine being imposed.
Luxembourg	No proceedings take place if possession is for personal use.
Netherlands	Up to 5 grams of cannabis, or 12 cigarettes, can be purchased in the cafes for personal use.
Portugal	Possessing cannabis for personal use is being decriminalized.
Spain	Using cannabis for personal use has been decriminalized and replaced by administrative sanctions.
Sweden	Personal users are offered counselling, but if they refuse to cooperate a fine is imposed.
UK	Possession of cannabis for personal use usually results in a formal warning or caution. A formal caution remains on police records for five years.

Footnote

It is extremely unlikely that the Prison Service would allow prisoners to have cannabis in possession were decriminalization to occur, for the following reasons:

(a) allowing the possession of cannabis for personal use would cause prison staff enormous difficulties in trying to control the activities of drug dealers and those involved in smuggling drugs into prisons;

(b) cannabis would become another form of currency in prisons alongside tobacco;

(c) cannabis can present special risks for those with mental health problems;

(d) a significant number of prisoners have mental health and alcohol-related problems;

(e) alcohol is not permitted in prisons (although it can be legally consumed by anyone over the age of 18);

(f) although decriminalizing cannabis means the law is prepared to tolerate its use under certain circumstances, it still remains illegal;

(g) cannabis is not socially acceptable in the UK and to permit its use would be politically unacceptable and contrary to the Government's drug policy at the present time;

(h) cannabis use is inconsistent with the promotion of healthy lifestyles.

Glossary

Addiction is the compulsive use of a drug and is a chronic condition. It causes physical, social and psychological problems for which there are no known cures. Relapse problems can arise at any time as addicts frequently require further treatment.

Chemical deterrence Opiate dependence can be treated by trexan (Naltrexone). This drug interferes with the receptivity of the brain to heroin and stops it having any effect on the individual.

Chemotherapy This is where chemicals are used to treat cancer and the debilitating symptoms and side effects of a life-threatening illness. Methadone treatment involves substituting methadone for more harmful opiates such as heroin, as legitimate clinical practice.

Dependence When a drug is taken over a lengthy period of time, the body adapts to its presence in the body. Once the user stops taking the drug the body reacts with withdrawal symptoms. Dependence is treated by gradually withdrawing the drug over a period of time.

Detoxification This is the process by which addicts gradually withdraw from the drug they are addicted to under medical supervision. Sometimes this can be achieved using other less harmful drugs, as is the case with heroin addiction.

Intoxication describes how a drug affects the individual physically and psychologically. The effects of drugs can vary but are generally short-lived because the drug is rapidly broken down chemically in the body and eventually excreted. High doses can take several days to process and, if the quantity taken is excessive and overloads the body's coping mechanism, coma and death can result.

Methadone Heroin addicts undergoing detoxification are given methadone prescriptions and counselling. Users can be accepted on a reduction programme where the ultimate goal is to achieve total abstinence. Another option is a maintenance programme, which tries to minimize the impact of drug misuse on individuals and helps them to give up a self-destructive lifestyle. This programme also tackles social, physical and psychological problems connected with drug dependency.

Overdose Taking an overdose can lead to coma or death. An antidote exists for some drugs which counteracts the effects of the poison in the body. There is no antidote for other drugs and treatment consists of maintaining the body's essential life support systems until the drug has cleared from the body. Adulterated drugs often complicate the problem of dealing with overdosing and is common in many of the street drugs smuggled into penal establishments.

Relapse   Prevention is the aim of most drug agencies. It is a regular occurrence with addicts who return to using drugs and then feel guilty for letting others down. Often they try to hide the fact that they have begun taking drugs again.

Sobriety   This is the condition achieved following abstinence and implies a lasting change to an individual's lifestyle, values, attitudes and behaviour. Sobriety is the closest to a cure that can ever be achieved.

The twelve steps programme   was originally devised by Alcoholics Anonymous in 1930 and published in their handbook called the *Big Book*. The twelve steps programme has been adapted by other self-help groups such as Gamblers Anonymous and Cocaine Anonymous. It has been used successfully by the Rehabilitation for Addicted Prisoners Trust (RAPt) at HMP Downview (see Chapter 8). The original twelve steps programme was set down as follows:

1. We admitted we were powerless over alcohol; that our lives had become unmanageable.
2. Came to believe that a Power greater than ourselves could restore us to sanity.
3. Make a decision to turn our will and our lives over to the care of God as we understood Him.
4. Make a searching and fearless moral inventory of ourselves.
5. Admitted to God, to ourselves and another human being the exact nature of our wrongs.
6. Were entirely ready to have God remove our shortcomings.
7. Humbly asked Him to remove our shortcomings.
8. Made a list of all persons we had harmed, and became willing to make amends to them all.
9. Made direct amends to such people wherever possible, except when to do so would injure them or others.
10. Continued to take personal inventory and when we were wrong promptly admitted it.
11. Sought through prayer and mediation to improve our conscious contact with God as we understood Him, praying only for knowledge of His will for us and the power to carry that out.
12. Having had a spiritual awakening as the result of these Steps, we tried to carry this message to others, and to practice these principles in all our affairs.

Tolerance   The body adapts to regular use of a drug so that larger and larger doses are needed to achieve the same effect. The danger of compensating by increasing the dose is the risk of overdosing.

Withdrawal   This term is used to describe the process for treating drug dependence. It involves gradually reducing the drug dose over a period of time in order to counter the severe side effects of drug addiction.

APPENDIX I

Documents

MANDATORY DRUG TEST AUTHORISATION FORM

Prisoner Name: .... Number: ....

Test Reference Number:

For allocation when sample is collected

1. The governor has authorised that in accordance with Section 16A of the Prison Act 1952 any prisoner may be required by a prison officer to provide a sample of urine for the purposes of testing for the presence of a controlled drug.

2. You are now required under the terms of Section 16A to provide a fresh and unadulterated sample of urine for testing for the presence of controlled drugs.

3. Authority for this requirement was given by: ....

4. Reason for requirement: (only one box to be ticked)

    [ ] **Random test:** You have been selected for this test on a strictly random basis.

    [ ] **Reasonable suspicion:** You have been selected for this test because staff have reason to believe that you have misused drugs. This test has been approved by a senior manager.

    [ ] **Risk assessment:** You have been selected for this test because you are being considered for a privilege, or a job, where a high degree of trust is to be given to you.

    [ ] **Frequent test programme:** You have been selected for more frequent testing because of your previous history of drug misuse.

    [ ] **On reception:** You have been selected for testing on reception on a random basis.

5. The procedures used during the collection and testing of the sample have been designed to protect you and to ensure that there are no mistakes in the handling of your sample. At the end of the collection procedure you will be asked to sign a statement confirming that the urine sealed in the sample bottles for testing is fresh and your own.

6. Your sample will be split at the point of collection into separate containers which will be sealed in your presence. In the event of you disputing any positive test result, one of these containers will be available, for a period of up to 12 months, for you to arrange, if you so wish, for an independent analysis to be undertaken at your own expense.

7. You will be liable to be placed on report if you:

    (a) provide a positive sample;
    (b) refuse to provide a sample; or,
    (c) fail to provide a sample after 4 hours of the order to do so (or after 5 hours if the officer believes that you are experiencing real difficulty in providing a sample).

Consent to Medical disclosure

   * (i)   During the past 30 days I have not used any medication issued to me by Health Care.

   * (ii) During the past 30 days I have used medication issued to me by Health Care. I understand that some medication issued by Health Care may affect the result of the test. I give my consent to the Medical Officer to provide details of this treatment to the prison authorities.

(*Delete as appropriate)

Signature of Prisoner : .... Date: ....

MDTA/12/95

PRISON SERVICE CHAIN OF CUSTODY PROCEDURE

Prisoner Name: ....   Number: ....

NON-RANDOM TESTING PROGRAMME (Tick box on tear-off section to indicate reason for test)

Checklist for sample collection - tick boxes as you proceed. Refer to guidance notes if in doubt.

1 [ ] Only **One** sample collection kit present.
2 [ ] Check identity of prisoner. Complete details above and in sample collection register.
3 [ ] Carry out search and handwashing procedures (No soap).
4 [ ] Show the prisoner that the collection cup and bottles are empty.
5 [ ] Ask prisoner to provide enough urine to be split **equally** between the two sample bottles.
6 [ ] *When a temperature check is necessary, take temperature using a thermometer or temperature strip in accordance with the supplier's instructions. If temperature is out of range (32-38C) (90-100F), make note in comments section and refer to guidance notes.*
7 [ ] **Watched by prisoner,** transfer urine **equally** between the two bottles. **Press caps on securely.**
8 [ ] Ask prisoner to initial and date both bottle seals.
9 [ ] **Watched by prisoner,** place a seal over each bottle cap.
10 [ ] Dispose of any surplus urine and the cup.
11 [ ] Pack two bottles in mailing container and then in chain of custody bag - **Do not seal bag.**
12 [ ] **Watched by prisoner,** fix barcode labels and enter test reference number on all copies of this form.
13 [ ] Ask the prisoner to sign and date the Prisoner's Declaration below.
14 [ ] Complete Chain of Custody Report, tear off and place in chain of custody bag facing outwards.
15 [ ] Seal bag, ask prisoner to initial bag where indicated.
16 [ ] Place sealed bag in secure refrigerator until ready for despatch to laboratory.
17 [ ] Allow prisoner to leave.

Prisoner Declaration

I confirm that (i)   I understand why I was required to provide the sample and what may happen if I fail to comply with this requirement;
           (ii) the urine sample I have given was my own and freshly provided;
           (iii) the sample was divided into two bottles and sealed in my presence with seals initialled and dated by me;
           (iv) the seals used on these bottles carry a barcode identical to the barcode attached to this form.

Signature of prisoner ....   Date ....

(Tear off along perforation)

Comments

CHAIN OF CUSTODY REPORT

Reason for test *(tick 1 box):*   [ ] Suspicion: [ ] Frequent: [ ] Reception: [ ] Risk:

Collecting officer declaration

Name (Print) ....   Prison ....
I confirm that the enclosed sample, bearing the Barcode identified below, was collected in accordance with the sample collection procedures agreed between the Prison Service and the laboratory.

Prisoner's Sex *(tick 1 box)* [ ]M   [ ]F   Prisoner's Ethnic Code..................................   Test Reference Number:

Sample collected on Date ....   Time ....

Signature of Collecting officer ....   Barcode

For the information of the laboratory only

[ ]   **NON RANDOM**

For laboratory use only

Name .... Signature .... Date .... Time ....

MDTLN/4/96

APPENDIX II

Addresses

This section contains a selection of useful organizations involved in helping those with drug dependency problems, and drug service providers to penal establishments.

Acorn Community Drug and Alcohol Services, Frith Cottage, Church Road, Surrey GU16 5AD.
Telephone 01276-670883
A drug service provider to establishments.

Addaction, Central Office, 67–69 Cowcross Street, London EC1M 6PU.
Telephone 020 7251-5860
A drug service provider to establishments.

Adfam National, Waterbridge House, 32–36 Loman Street, London SE1 0EE.
Telephone 020 7928-8900
It runs a national helpline to support the families and friends of drug users.

Avon & West Wilts Mental Health NHS Trust, Robert Smith Unit, 12 Mortimer Road, Clifton, Bristol BS8 4EX.
Telephone 0117-973-5004
A drug service provider to establishments.

Cocaine Anonymous, telephone 020 7284-1123
Provides a helpline for cocaine users.

Compass, Kings House, 12 Kings Street, York YO1 9WP.
Telephone 01904-636374
A major drug service provider to establishments.

Cranstoun Drug Services, 4th Floor, Broadway House, 112–134 The Broadway, Wimbledon, London SW19 1RL.
Telephone 020 8543-8333
Provides a range of specialist drug treatment and rehabilitation services catering for users in residential accommodation, prisons and the community.

East Kent Community NHS Trust, Littlebourne Road, Canterbury, Kent CT1 1AZ.
Telephone 01227-459371
A drug service provider at an establishment.

Exeter Drug Project, Dean Clarke House, Southernhay East, Exeter EX1 1PQ.
Telephone 01392-666710
A drug service provider to establishments.

ISDD, Institute for the Study of Drug Dependence, 32–36 Loman Street, London SE1 0EE.
Telephone 020 7928-1211
Produces authoritative drug information in the form of leaflets, booklets and a bi-monthly magazine.

Kent Council on Addiction, DAN House, East Street, Faversham, Kent ME13 8AT.
Telephone 01795-590635
A drug service provider at an establishment.

Life for the World, Life for the World Trust, Wakefield Building, Gomm Road, High Wycombe, Bucks HP13 7DJ.
Telephone 01494-462008
A Christian-based organization committed to helping with the rehabilitation of drug addicts into the community.

Lifeline Project Ltd, c/o Psychology Department, HMP Wymott, Ulnes Walton Lane, Leyland, Lancashire PR5 3LW.
Telephone 01772-421461
A drug service provider to establishments.

Mind, telephone 020 8522-1728 and 0345-660163
Provides services for those suffering with mental health problems and drug users.

NACRO, National Association for the Care and Resettlement of Offenders, 169 Clapham Road, London SW9 0OU.
Telephone 020 7582-6500
Provides information for prisoners and their families on a wide range of matters, including drug services.

Narcotics Anonymous, telephone 020 7730-0009
Provides a telephone helpline for drug addicts.

National Aids Helpline, telephone 0800-567-123
Provides a 24-hour helpline to those concerned about AIDS/HIV.

National Drugs Helpline, telephone 0800-776600
Provides a 24-hour helpline and advice to anyone concerned about drug misuse.

Phoenix House, Phoenix House, 3rd Floor, Afra House, 1 Long Lane, London SE1 4PG.
Telephone 020 7234-9740
A drug service provider to establishments.

RAPt, Rehabilitation for Addicted Prisoners Trust, 179–181 Vauxhall Bridge Road, London SW1V 1ER.
Telephone 020 8976-6688
Provides 12-step drug rehabilitation programmes in penal establishments.

Release, 388 Old Street, London EC1V 9LT.
Telephone 020 7729-2599
Provides a 24-hour national legal and drug advice service.

Samaritans, telephone 0345-909090
Offers a 24-hour support and advice service to anyone in crisis and danger of self-harm.

Shropshire Community Substance Misuse Team, St. Michaels House, St Michaels Street, Shrewsbury SY1 2HG.
Telephone 01743-255741
A drug service provider at an establishment.

Terence Higgins Trust, telephone 020 7242-1010
Provides a helpline for anyone concerned about AIDS/HIV.

Trafford Substance Misuse Services, Chapel Road, Sale M33 7FD.
Telephone 0161-912-3170
A drug service provider to establishments.

Turning Point, New Loom House, 101 Backchurch Lane, London E1 1LU.
Telephone 020 7702-2300
A drug service provider to establishments.

Index

Active Drug Detection Dogs (ADDD) 41, 60
acceptance 118
accessibility 118
accreditation 111
Acquired Immune Deficiency Syndrome
    (AIDS) 106
adjudication guidelines 78
adulteration 3
Advisory Council on the Misuse of Drugs 35
Aftercare 142
All Party Parliamentary Drug Misuse
    Group 32, 35
amphetamines 5–6, 68
amphetamine sulphate 13
amylobarbitone 18
Annual Report 90
Area Drug Coordinators 28, 40
Area Manager 42
assault 63
Ativan 16
Attention Deficit Disorder (ADD) 115
attitude 118
auricular acupuncture 115
Austria 192

Bacillus Calmete-Guérin (BCG) 109
bail information 48, 120
barbiturates 5–6, 18, 68
basic regime 100
basic skills test 111
Belgium 193
benzodiazepine tranquillizers 5, 6
benzodiazepines 16, 68
Blind Performance Challenge Programme 71
blood spread 107
Board of Visitors (BoV) 42, 52
Britofex 114
butobarbitone 18

cannabis 6, 68
cannabis resin 5

cannabis sativa 6
CARAT assessment 82
CARAT services 45, 82
CARAT worker 85
care plans 46, 85
cassette 95
CCTV 26, 31, 55–6, 140
Chain of Custody procedure 68
chaplaincy team 42
chlorodiazepoxide 16
Class A drugs 4, 191
Class B drugs 5, 191
Class C drugs 5, 191
closed visits 52
cocaine 6, 11, 68
cocaine freebase 11
cocaine hydrochloride 12
codeine 5
coercion 53
Cognitive Skills programmes 123
cold turkey 9
community-based agencies 42
Community Drug Treatment services 130
community visits 101
compacts 96–7, 121
Comprehensive Spending Review (CSR) 29,
    45, 133
conduct reports 73
confidential telephone line 53
confidentiality 84, 118
confirmation test 69, 76
confirmation test report 69
controlled drug 75
Controller 72
counselling 46, 49, 116–18
Counselling, Assessment, Referral, Advice
    and Throughcare Service 25, 45
crack 11
Cranstoun Drug Services 93
credibility 118
crime reduction strategy 148

Criminal Justice Act 1991 125
Criminal Justice and Public Order Act 1994 66
crisis-intervention strategy 148
Crown Prosecution Service (CPS) 48

Dalmane 16
deaths in custody 30
decision-making counselling 117
decriminalization 191
dedicated drug worker 138
defence 74
denies access 64
Denmark 193
depression 119
detains any person 64
detoxification 91, 112
detropoxyphene 5
dexamphetamine 13
diacetymorphine 8
diamorphine 8
diazepam 16
diethypropion 5
dip and read testing 72, 94–5
Diploma in Achievement 111
Directorate of Regimes 40
disinfecting tablets 110
disciplinary action 72
Divisional Court 76
dog handlers 61
Drug Action Teams (DATs) 26
Drug and Alcohol Awareness 111
Drug and Alcohol Action Teams (DAATs) 26
drug amnesty bin 53
drug counselling 115–18
drug detection dogs 26
drug-free wings 91
'Drug Misuse in Prison' 39, 91
drug misuser profile 31
drug prevention 51
Drug Reference Groups (DRGs) 28
Drug Strategy 185
Drug Strategy Coordinator 41, 49, 136
Drug Strategy Team 43
Drug Strategy Unit 30
drug testing machine 93
Drug Trafficking Act 1994 5
'drug tsar' 141
drug treatment programmes 131

ecstasy 6, 15
education contractor 42
electronic detection devices 55
enhanced earnings scheme 101
enhanced regime 102

Enzyme Multiplied Immunoassay Technique (EMIT) 93
escapes 64
Euromed 95
European Convention of Human Rights 52

fights 64
Finland 193
flurazepam 16
forward planning 187
France 193
freebasing 13
frequent drug-testing programme 53, 67
full assessment 46
future developments 189

Gas Chromatography/Mass Spectometry (GC/MS) 69
Germany 193
Good Order and Discipline (GOAD) 35
Governor 41, 72
Greece 192
groupwork 46, 49, 123

hallucinogenic amphetamines 15
hallucinogens 4
health care 46, 186
health care staff 106
health education 110
Hellawell, Keith 55, 141
hepatitis 44
hepatitis B 108
hepatitis C 109
herbal cannabis 8
Her Majesty's Chief Inspector of Prisons (HMCIP) 29, 151
heroin 8
HMP Bristol 161
HMP Exeter 169
HMP Highdown 160
HMP Liverpool 151
HMP Preston 173
HMP Wayland 178
HMP Wormwood Scrubs 156
HMP Wymott 154
HMP & HMYOI Hollesley Bay Colony 179
HMP & YOI Bullwood Hall 172
HMP & YOI Parc 166
HMYOI Hatfield 176
HMYOI Huntercombe 158
HMYOI & RC Reading 164
HIV anti-body test 107
Home Affairs Committee on Drugs and Prisons 55, 133, 138
Home Detention Curfew (HDC) 49

Home Office Drugs Prevention Teams 29
human imunodeficiency virus (HIV) 44, 106
Human Rights Act 144
hydrochloride 11
hypnotic drugs 5

Incentive and Earned Privilege Scheme
  (IEPS) 53, 99, 122
independent laboratory analysis 70
induction programmes 141
infected mother 107
Infexidine hydrochloride 114
'Information for Prisoners Who Have Tested
  Positive for Drugs' 76
informants 56
intelligence 53
intelligence-gathering 55
international dimension 190
Ireland 193

Joint Prison Health Care Task Force 105
Joint Prison Health Policy Unit 105

knowledge 118

laboratory 67
laboratory scientist 76
laevo-amphetamine 13
Learmont Report 31, 91
legal defences 75
Librium 16
London School of Hygiene & Tropical
  Medicine 110
lorazepam 16
LSD 6, 19, 68
Luxembourg 193
lysergic acid diethylamide (LSD) 6, 19, 68

Mandatory Drug Test Authorization Form 68
Mandatory Drug Testing (MDT) 5, 33, 142,
  187
mandatory frequent testing 79
mecloqualone 5
Medical Officer 73
Medical Research Council (MRC) 6
Medicines Act 1968 3
meprobamate 5
methadone 6, 10, 68
methadone maintenance programmes 130
methadone reduction programmes 130
methaqualone 5
methylamphetamine 13
methylene-dioxy-methyl-amphetamine
  (MDMA) 15
methylphenidate 5, 13

Minnesota twelve-steps programme 93, 121
Misuse of Drugs Act 1971 4, 35
mitigating circumstances 73
Mogadon 16
multi-disciplinary approach 45
multi-disciplinary framework 85
multi-disciplinary team 42
multiple screening tests 96
Mycobacterium tuberculosis 109

naltrexone 113
National Curriculum Framework 110
National Health Service (NHS) 26
National Policy Framework 99
National Treatment Outcome Research
  Study 129
needs assessment 43
Nembutal 18
Netherlands 193
nitrazepam 16
Normison 16

Observation Classification and Allocation
  (OCA) 84
offences against discipline 63
Office for National Statistics 105
ongoing support 118
Open College 93
Operational Standards 61
opiates 4, 6, 68
opium poppy 8
orientation 12
oxazepam 16
Oxford Centre for Criminalogical Research 33

Passive Drug Detection Dogs (PDDD) 41, 60,
  140
pentazocine 5
pentobarbitone 18
performance targets 25
pharmacy medicines 3
phencyclidine 4
phenobarbital 68
phentermine 5
physeptone 10, 113
police liaison officer 44
Portugal 193
post-release 86
pregnancy 2
pre-release courses 124, 136
prescribed drugs 58
prescription only 3
Primary Intervention programmes 144
primary treatment 122
prison link officers 136

Prison Rules 1999 51, 63, 66
'Prisons and Drug Misuse' report 35
probation officers 136
probation team 42
problem-solving counselling 118
professional competence 118
'Protecting the Public' 105
psychiatric disorders 118
psychology department 42
punishments 77

quinalbarbitone 5, 18

Ramsbotham, Sir David 30
random drug testing 58, 67
random searching of staff 139
reasonable doubt 75
reasonable suspicion 67
Reasoning and Rehabilitation
    programme 123
reception 46, 67, 185
'Reducing Crime' 105
rehabilitation programmes 25
release plan 86
remand prisoners 86
research 133, 142
risk assessment 67
rohypnol 5
rub down search 52

schizophrenia 119
screening test 69
seamless throughcare 138
Seconal 18
security department 42
Security Information Report (SIR) 46
sedatives 5
segregation units 139
Self-Harm at Risk form 84
self-help groups 121
self-inflicted deaths 30
sentence management 136
sentenced prisoners 88
Serenid 16
SMART targets 85
smuggling drugs 52–3
Social and Life Skills 111
Soneryl 18
staff training 91, 189
standard regime 101

Standards Audit Team 145
Standards Audit Unit 145–6
Standards Manual 99
substance abuse 30
Substance Abuse and Mental Health Services
    Administration (SAMHSA) 95
'Suicide is Everyone's Concern' 30
supply of drugs 43
Sweden 193
Syva/EMIT systems 94

'Tackling Drugs to Build a Better Britain' 22,
    25, 39
'Tackling Drugs in Prison' 28, 39, 90
'Tackling Drugs Together' 22
targeted mandatory drug-testing 59
temazepam 5, 16
tetrahydrocannabinol 6
therapeutic communities 91, 120–1, 129
Thinking Skills programme 124
throughcare 91, 133, 136, 186
toxins 112
treatment 85, 127
treatment programmes 120, 140
tuberculosis (TB) 109
Tuinal 18

UK 192
UK Anti-Drugs Coordinator 25, 55
unauthorized item 51
unprotected sexual intercourse 107
urine-based immunoassay screening test 95
urine sample 68

Valium 16
Viagra 16
visitors 51
Visitors Centre 53, 140
voluntary drug testing 94
Voluntary Testing Unit (VTU) 30, 91–2

withdrawal 113
women 46
Woolf Report 1991 91, 96

Young Offenders Institution (YOI) 44
YOI Rules 1999 63

zero tolerance 35